EMERGENCY AND INTENSIVE CARE MEDICINE

PERITONITIS

CAUSES, DIAGNOSIS AND TREATMENT

DAVID F. WALKER
EDITOR

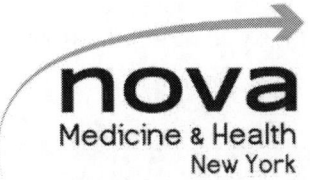

Copyright © 2021 by Nova Science Publishers, Inc.

All rights reserved. No part of this book may be reproduced, stored in a retrieval system or transmitted in any form or by any means: electronic, electrostatic, magnetic, tape, mechanical photocopying, recording or otherwise without the written permission of the Publisher.

We have partnered with Copyright Clearance Center to make it easy for you to obtain permissions to reuse content from this publication. Simply navigate to this publication's page on Nova's website and locate the "Get Permission" button below the title description. This button is linked directly to the title's permission page on copyright.com. Alternatively, you can visit copyright.com and search by title, ISBN, or ISSN.

For further questions about using the service on copyright.com, please contact:
Copyright Clearance Center
Phone: +1-(978) 750-8400　　　　　Fax: +1-(978) 750-4470　　　　　E-mail: info@copyright.com.

NOTICE TO THE READER

The Publisher has taken reasonable care in the preparation of this book, but makes no expressed or implied warranty of any kind and assumes no responsibility for any errors or omissions. No liability is assumed for incidental or consequential damages in connection with or arising out of information contained in this book. The Publisher shall not be liable for any special, consequential, or exemplary damages resulting, in whole or in part, from the readers' use of, or reliance upon, this material. Any parts of this book based on government reports are so indicated and copyright is claimed for those parts to the extent applicable to compilations of such works.

Independent verification should be sought for any data, advice or recommendations contained in this book. In addition, no responsibility is assumed by the Publisher for any injury and/or damage to persons or property arising from any methods, products, instructions, ideas or otherwise contained in this publication.

This publication is designed to provide accurate and authoritative information with regard to the subject matter covered herein. It is sold with the clear understanding that the Publisher is not engaged in rendering legal or any other professional services. If legal or any other expert assistance is required, the services of a competent person should be sought. FROM A DECLARATION OF PARTICIPANTS JOINTLY ADOPTED BY A COMMITTEE OF THE AMERICAN BAR ASSOCIATION AND A COMMITTEE OF PUBLISHERS.

Additional color graphics may be available in the e-book version of this book.

Library of Congress Cataloging-in-Publication Data

Names: Walker, David F. (Nova Publishers editor) editor.
Title: Peritonitis : causes, diagnosis and treatment / David F. Walker,
　editor.
Description: New York : Nova Science Publishers, [2021] | Series: Emergency
　and intensive care medicine | Includes bibliographical references and
　index. |
Identifiers: LCCN 2021019810 (print) | LCCN 2021019811 (ebook) | ISBN
　9781536196245 (paperback) | ISBN 9781536196412 (adobe pdf)
Subjects: LCSH: Peritonitis.
Classification: LCC RC867 .P483 2021 (print) | LCC RC867 (ebook) | DDC
　618.7/4--dc23
LC record available at https://lccn.loc.gov/2021019810
LC ebook record available at https://lccn.loc.gov/2021019811

Published by Nova Science Publishers, Inc. † New York

CONTENTS

Preface		**vii**
Chapter 1	Postoperative Peritonitis – The Burden of Complicated Intraabdominal Infection Management *Manol B. Sokolov and Dochka T. Tzoneva*	**1**
Chapter 2	Peritonitis in Assisted Peritoneal Dialysis. Results of a Consolidated Program *Consolación Rosado-Rubio, Isabelle Brayer, Carla Bernaer, Nadine Rossez, Elena Vieru, Christelle Fosso and Max Dratwa*	**69**
Chapter 3	Secondary Peritonitis: Causes, Diagnosis and Treatment *Carlos San Miguel-Méndez, Jaime Ruiz-Tovar, Ana Minaya-Bravo, Marina Perez-Flecha and Miguel Angel Garcia-Ureña*	**87**
Index		**103**

PREFACE

This book contains three chapters about peritonitis, which is an inflammation of the membrane lining the abdominal wall and covering the abdominal organs. Chapter one presents classification of postoperative peritonitis, describes symptoms, reviews the current understanding of the phases and stages of development and features of the disease, and discusses the usefulness of different prognostic scales for assessment of complicated intra-abdominal infections. Chapter two studies assisted peritoneal dialysis, wherein a nurse goes to the patient's home to perform the dialysis technique when the patient is unable to do it himself. Chapter three discusses in detail different types of peritoneum infections, including their principles of diagnosis and treatment options.

Chapter 1 - *Introduction.* Complicated intra-abdominal infections (cIAIs) are an important cause of morbidity and mortality. Despite advances in modern surgery, intensive care, imaging methods, specific clinical, laboratory, and immunological markers, the timely diagnosis of postoperative peritonitis remains difficult. Its complex management requires huge resources with often adverse outcome, regardless of the joint efforts of the multidisciplinary team. *Material and Methods.* In this publication, the authors present classification of postoperative peritonitis, description of symptoms, review the current understanding of the phases and stages of development, and features of the disease, and the authors also discuss the usefulness of different prognostic scales for assessment of cIAIs. Based on the contemporary knowledge in medical science, the authors present modern guidelines for the diagnosis and treatment of cIAIs. The authors pay special attention to the preoperative preparation, surgical remediation timing, options for completion of the primary operation (closed method, relaparotomy "on demand" or "planned," or laparostomy), and further determination of patient management tactics, postoperative complications (enterocutaneous fistula formation, abscesses, upper gastrointestinal mucosal stress-related injury, abdominal compartment syndrome, wound infection, thromboembolic and pulmonary complications), as well as current challenges related to the treatment of infections caused by multidrug-resistant pathogens. The authors present their own experience at retrospective analysis of postoperative peritonitis cases in the Department of Surgery/Intensive Care Unit at University Hospital Alexandrovska, Sofia for the last ten years. *Results.* Development of postoperative peritonitis - associated with penetration into the peritoneal cavity - has been found in 64 adult patients out of 4943 surgeries (1.29%) (33 male and 31 female aged from 29 to 92 years) for the period from 2011 to 2020. Tertiary generalized peritonitis was found in 24 patients; and there has been more than one relaparotomy in 18 patients. The etiology of postoperative peritonitis in the authors' patients is quite diverse, and the most cases were due to insufficiency of the anastomosis (29 cases), dehiscence of the surgical wound (22), iatrogenic lesion of the viscera (4), and necrotizing pancreatitis (3). The authors observed a mortality rate of 39% in their cohort. Relaparotomy has been performed in a wide range of times after primary surgery - from 1st to 15th postoperative day in protracted cases; planned relaparotomy - in 14 patients ended with laparostomy, and subsequent "conducting" with staged reexplorations; "on demand" relaparotomy - in 50 patients; laparostomy with negative pressure therapy – in 12 patients. *Conclusion.* Development of postoperative peritonitis continues to be a life-threatening complication. Mortality is determined by the inability of radical control of the septic source in connection with persistent septic abdomen, advanced age, poor performance status (higher APACHE II score), and unreasonably delayed relaparotomy. The main factors in the effective treatment of cIAIs are: (1) rapid diagnosis and identification of high-risk patients; (2) adequate resuscitation; (3) early initiation of appropriate antibiotic therapy; (4) early and effective control of the source of infection; and (5) reassessment of the clinical response and appropriate adjustment of the therapeutic strategy. The authors adhere to the opinion that more aggressive treatment approach could reduce the mortality/morbidity rate and the decision for prompt ("early") relaparotomy is crucial in treatment of generalized postoperative peritonitis.

Chapter 2 - Peritoneal dialysis is a main part of the treatment of the end-stage kidney disease. It offers results comparable to hemodialysis. It provides a home dialysis treatment, which offers some advantages in order to improve the patient's quality of life, mainly in elderly people. One of the most serious complications is peritonitis, which can lead to the technique failure and the patient's transfer to hemodialysis. Assisted peritoneal dialysis is a peritoneal dialysis modality in which a nurse goes to the patient's home to perform the dialysis technique when the patient is unable to do it himself (elderly or disabled people) and there is a lack of family support. The authors have studied the assisted peritoneal dialysis program of the CHU Brugmann, in Brussels, a consolidated program who was implemented many years ago, in order to know its organization, the way of performing the technique and the rate of peritonitis in this kind of peritoneal dialysis since the implantation of the technique in the hospital. Assisted peritoneal dialysis in CHU Brugmann is supported by home-care companies, who provide the visiting nurses. The hospital has imposed a very strict training protocol to the visiting nurses, so the rate of peritonitis is weak (not superior to autonomous patients or patients helped by their family). Assisted peritoneal dialysis in hospitals who have a consolidated program is a safe and valid way of performing an in-home treatment of the end-stage chronic kidney to avoid the transfer to hemodialysis in a sanitary facility.

Chapter 3 - The peritoneum is a semipermeable membrane that allows a flux of solutes into and from the peritoneal cavity. Peritonitis denotes inflammation of the peritoneum, whose cause is not specific. It mainly exists two different types of this intraabdominal infection: spontaneous bacterial peritonitis (SBP) or secondary peritonitis (SP). SPB is often presented in cirrhotic patients, in whom altered small intestinal motility and the presence of hypochlorhydria due to the use of proton pump inhibitors predisposes an overgrowth of specific organisms, especially *E. Coli*. They are those processes in which a source of intra-abdominal contamination cannot be evidenced. In SP, the infection is produced by the breakdown of the anatomo-functional barrier of the wall of the gastrointestinal tract or annex glands, with a discharge of septic content into the peritoneal cavity. The main causes are the following: acute appendicitis, diverticulitis, perforated peptic ulcer, intestinal obstruction with strangulation of the small bowel, trauma, pelvic infections and intraoperative contamination. SP is usually polymicrobial, with a predominance of gram-negative bacilli (such as *E. Coli* or *Klebsiella*) and anaerobic organisms (e.g., *Bacteroides fragilis*). Despite the advances in surgical techniques, antibiotic-therapy and intensive care support; mortality and morbidity remain high, while its management stays difficult and complex. In this chapter, the authors will discuss in detail these different types of peritoneum infections, with their principles of diagnosis and last evidence in treatment.

In: Peritonitis
Editor: David F. Walker

ISBN: 978-1-53619-624-5
© 2021 Nova Science Publishers, Inc.

Chapter 1

POSTOPERATIVE PERITONITIS – THE BURDEN OF COMPLICATED INTRAABDOMINAL INFECTION MANAGEMENT

Manol B. Sokolov[1,], MD, PhD and Dochka T. Tzoneva[2], MD, PhD*

[1]Department of Surgery, University Hospital Alexandrovska, Medical University Sofia, Bulgaria
[2]Clinic of Anaesthesia and Intensive Care, University Hospital Alexandrovska, Medical University, Sofia, Bulgaria

ABSTRACT

Introduction

Complicated intra-abdominal infections (cIAIs) are an important cause of morbidity and mortality. Despite advances in modern surgery,

---

[*] Corresponding Author's E-mail: m69sokolov@abv.bg; m6sokolov@gmail.com.

intensive care, imaging methods, specific clinical, laboratory, and immunological markers, the timely diagnosis of postoperative peritonitis remains difficult. Its complex management requires huge resources with often adverse outcome, regardless of the joint efforts of the multidisciplinary team.

Material and Methods

In this publication, we present classification of postoperative peritonitis, description of symptoms, review the current understanding of the phases and stages of development, and features of the disease, and we also discuss the usefulness of different prognostic scales for assessment of cIAIs. Based on the contemporary knowledge in medical science, we present modern guidelines for the diagnosis and treatment of cIAIs. We pay special attention to the preoperative preparation, surgical remediation timing, options for completion of the primary operation (closed method, relaparotomy "on demand" or "planned," or laparostomy), and further determination of patient management tactics, postoperative complications (enterocutaneous fistula formation, abscesses, upper gastrointestinal mucosal stress-related injury, abdominal compartment syndrome, wound infection, thromboembolic and pulmonary complications), as well as current challenges related to the treatment of infections caused by multidrug-resistant pathogens. We present our own experience at retrospective analysis of postoperative peritonitis cases in the Department of Surgery/Intensive Care Unit at University Hospital Alexandrovska, Sofia for the last ten years.

Results

Development of postoperative peritonitis - associated with penetration into the peritoneal cavity - has been found in 64 adult patients out of 4943 surgeries (1.29%) (33 male and 31 female aged from 29 to 92 years) for the period from 2011 to 2020. Tertiary generalized peritonitis was found in 24 patients; and there has been more than one relaparotomy in 18 patients. The etiology of postoperative peritonitis in our patients is quite diverse, and the most cases were due to insufficiency of the anastomosis (29 cases), dehiscence of the surgical wound (22), iatrogenic lesion of the viscera (4), and necrotizing pancreatitis (3). We observed a mortality rate of 39% in our cohort. Relaparotomy has been performed in a wide range of times after primary surgery - from 1st to 15th postoperative day in protracted cases; planned relaparotomy - in 14 patients ended with laparostomy, and subsequent "conducting" with staged reexplorations; "on demand" relaparotomy - in 50 patients; laparostomy with negative pressure therapy – in 12 patients.

Conclusion

Development of postoperative peritonitis continues to be a life-threatening complication. Mortality is determined by the inability of radical control of the septic source in connection with persistent septic abdomen, advanced age, poor performance status (higher APACHE II score), and unreasonably delayed relaparotomy. The main factors in the effective treatment of cIAIs are: (1) rapid diagnosis and identification of high-risk patients; (2) adequate resuscitation; (3) early initiation of appropriate antibiotic therapy; (4) early and effective control of the source of infection; and (5) reassessment of the clinical response and appropriate adjustment of the therapeutic strategy. We adhere to the opinion that more aggressive treatment approach could reduce the mortality/morbidity rate and the decision for prompt ("early") relaparotomy is crucial in treatment of generalized postoperative peritonitis.

Keywords: postoperative peritonitis, abdominal sepsis, relaparotomy, laparostomy, intensive care

INTRODUCTION

Despite the advance of modern surgery, intensive care, imaging methods, the adopted score systems for assessment, and specific clinical, laboratory, and immunological markers, the timely diagnostics of postoperative peritonitis remains difficult, while its complex management requires enormous resource with not infrequently unfavorable outcome, regardless of the joint efforts of the multidisciplinary team. The generalized postoperative peritonitis is defined as presence of inflammatory exudate and inflammatory changes over the visceral and parietal peritoneum with positive microbiological cultures, biliary or intestinal content in the four abdominal quadrants, found in the first month after abdominal operation, which was not performed due to peritonitis or abdominal trauma (secondary postoperative peritonitis), or due to primarily preceding peritonitis (tertiary postoperative peritonitis). "Early relaparotomy" is performed in the first 24 hours after the onset of infectious and inflammatory peritoneal pathological changes, while "late relaparotomy" – the one in which the delay is more than 24 hours after the complication occurrence.

The secondary peritonitis represents approximately 90% of all cases of peritonitis in the Western countries. Within this group the diffuse postoperative peritonitis (PP) and the abdominal sepsis are interconnected problems in consequence to surgical interventions. The modern literature demonstrates percentage between 30 and 42% for diffuse postoperative peritonitis in the subgroup of secondary peritonitis [1, 2]. Despite the advance of antibiotic therapy, and significant improvement in the intensive care, the morbidity (incidence) is high and mortality remains between 30% and 66% [3, 4].

The postoperative peritonitis is one of the most serious complications in the abdominal surgery. This contrasts with the small number of publications regarding this condition. The intra abdominal infections is most frequently a result of invasion and multiplication of intestinal bacteria in/through the wall of gastrointestinal tract (GIT). The generalized postoperative peritonitis is defined as presence of inflammatory exudate, and inflammatory changes over the visceral and parietal peritoneum, with positive microbiological cultures, biliary or intestinal content in the four abdominal quadrants, which was found in the first month after abdominal surgery, not performed due to peritonitis or abdominal trauma (secondary postoperative peritonitis), or due to primarily preceding peritonitis (tertiary postoperative peritonitis).

The invasive radiological manipulations and the modern aggressive antibiotics have improved the results regarding the postoperative abdominal abscesses, but the high mortality continues to be observed in patients with postoperative diffuse peritonitis. The postoperative diffuse peritonitis is a potentially life-threatening condition, and it is usually caused by leaking of intestinal content. Among the other causes are external intraoperative contamination, dissemination of residual infection, intestinal ischemia, postoperative peritonitis, etc. The cause is not always poor operative technique or wrong decision on the part of surgeon, but also the primary pathology, virulence of microorganisms, overall condition of patient during the first operation within the operative and postoperative therapeutic course of patient – all of which are playing a significant role.

The diagnostics of postoperative peritonitis is based mostly on clinical signs. Diagnostic characteristics are newly occurred or worsening abdominal pain (95%), ballooning of abdomen (75%), febricity (80%), tachycardia (95%) with physical (found upon palpation) data of irritation of the peritoneum (tenderness upon palpation; muscular defence to an extent of rigidity; positive Blumberg's sign) – (90%) in the postoperative period.

The tachypnea and hypotension are factors of poor prognosis. 100% mortality was registered among patients, who developed hypotension that is refractory to therapy.

Nausea, vomiting, increase of the secretion from the nasogastric tube – spontaneous or upon aspiration (90%); discontinuation of flatus and defecation (80%) with abdominal swelling suggest paralytic ileus due to peritonitis. Important signal sign is the pathological secretion from the surgical wound or drainages (75%) (small intestinal, feculent, biliary, or purulent), which is an indication for intraperitoneal leaking of content from gastrointestinal/biliary tract or residual peritonitis.

We demonstrated - in our study - that the regularly used clinical and laboratory parameters have limited predictive value in the diagnosis of postoperative peritonitis, compared to the group of patients with non-postoperative "acquired in the community" secondary peritonitis. A little more than 50% of patients in the group with postoperative peritonitis present with abdominal pain or sensitivity to palpation, accompanied with high temperature during the physical examination. And what is more, the clinical signs of peritonitis as muscular defence or positive Blumberg's sign are evident only in about 22% of these patients. This can be explained by the prevailing postaggressive catabolism, as well as by the postoperative administration of analgesics [7]. That is why these patients are frequently diagnosed, when the signs of sepsis have already occurred.

The low accuracy of the physical tests in diagnosis making of postoperative peritonitis reflects the dubious worth of surgeon's experience. Of course, the clinical assessment remains important, but, as it seems, it frequently fails in the setting of effective postoperative analgesia and sedation of intubated patients. The results from physical tests are not particularly important parameters in the determination of mortality of patients with relaparotomies, as a result of peritonitis, i.e., the physical tests do not provide meaningful variables regarding the prognosis of the occurring or continuing abdominal sepsis.

The methods for reduction of bacterial contamination of the first laparotomy for peritonitis were extensively discussed [9]. Two surgical strategies were adopted: relaparotomy "on indications"- on-demand relaparotomy (ODR); or elective relaparotomy – planned relaparotomy (PR). The approach of ODR is still, to a great extent, the most frequently used, even for severe peritonitis [10, 11]. By means of this approach, the difficult timely establishment of relapses or persisting symptoms of peritonitis [12] result in therapeutic delay, with multi organ failure and high mortality [13-15, 16-20]. In order the result to be improved, many authors defend the PR-approach as the proper one in patients with severe advanced peritonitis [21-24]. Retrospective studies [24-26] as well as results from a series of non-randomized prospective study [13], comparing PR and ODR, decrease the clinical and statistically significant benefit for survival in the PR approach after univariate analysis. On the contrary, two studies, which compare PR and ODR in a mixed series of mild and severe peritonitis [11, 23] do not find better survival after PR. It is possible that in the latter studies, disadvantages of PR in mild cases to result from the possibility of easy iatrogenic impairment of edematous tissues of visceral organs [24] and the subsequent aggravation of the systemic inflammatory reaction [25], neutralizing the advantages of PR in severe cases. In fact, the PR approach must be limited to the subgroup of patients with high risk of continuing intraabdominal infection. Based on our ascertainment, we recommend PR for postoperative generalized feculent peritonitis, which has a risk of 41% for continuous peritonitis, as well as for patients with uncertain control of the source of sepsis. We do not agree with the recommendation that all patients with postoperative peritonitis [26] or all patients with severe form of purulent peritonitis [27] must be subject to PR: after adequate initial control of the source of sepsis, only 9% of patients with postoperative generalized purulent, feculent, or biliary peritonitis develop recurrent sepsis.

Etiology

Leaking of intestinal content or bile juice after the initial laparotomy is the main cause for postoperative abdominal infection.

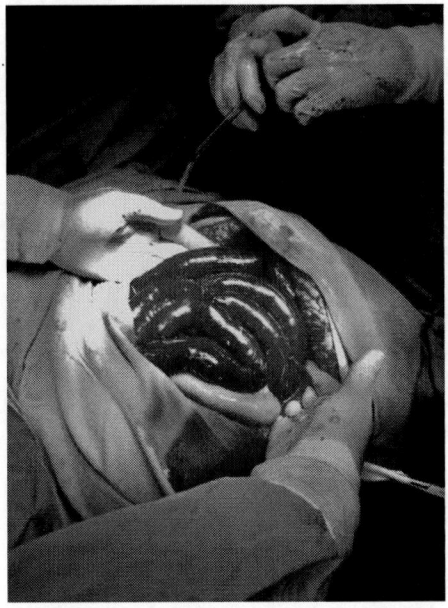

Figure 1. Peritonitis caused by intestinal ischemia.

Other causes include:

- residual contamination
- intestinal ischemia (Figure 1)

- de novo beginning of abdominal infection from a source not affected initially – postoperative pancreatitis, cholecystitis, perforation of the hollow organ etc. (Figure 2)
- dehiscence of the surgical wound with bacterial contamination (with/without infection at the surgical site – suppuration of the surgical wound) (Figure 3)

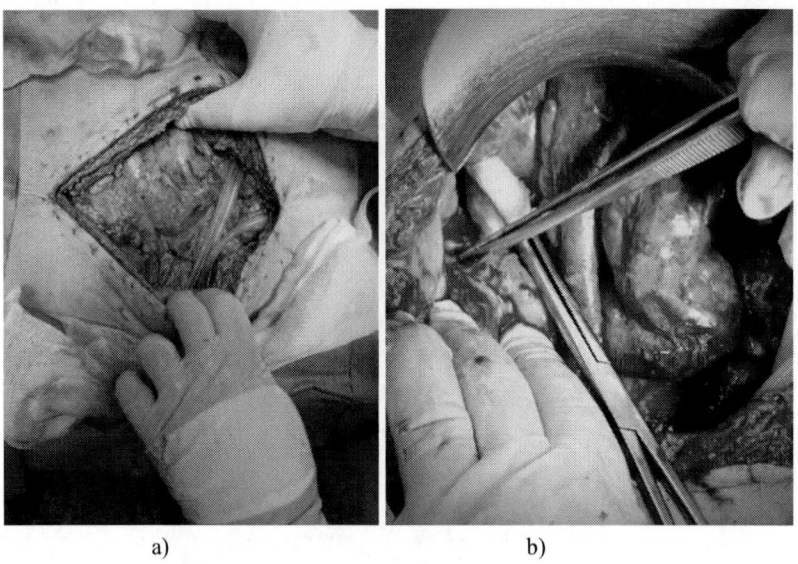

Figure 2. Peritonitis caused by postoperative perforation of the jejunum – a) intraoperative view in relaparotomy; b) jejunum perforation found as causative lesion.

The healing of the internal suture line or anastomoses depends on:

- The balance between lysis and synthesis of collagen. If the velocity of lysis exceeds the one of synthesis, even the evidently most fail-safe anastomoses can heal. This depends on the overall condition of patient, inclusively the nutritional state, which can be determined by measurement of parameters as serum albumin. It also depends on the presence of local infection.
- Techniques: technical disadvantages can be in the form of
  - Sutures placed too close to the cut end of visceral organ

- Sutures which do not include the submucous layer of intestines
- Present tension of the anastomosis
- The blood supply of the anastomosis is insufficient, in order to allow effective inflammatory reaction.
- The bacteria at the site of anastomosis cause acute inflammatory reaction and production of disintegrating neutrophil proteolytic enzymes, which destruct the intestinal tissue.
- Poor formation of serous membranes or passing through iatrogenic/pathological absence of serous membranes

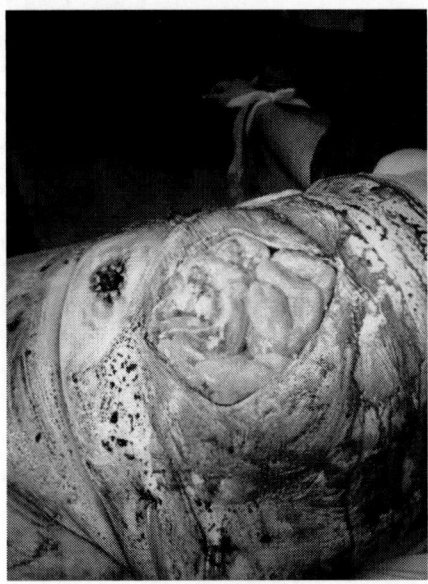

Figure 3. Peritonitis caused by surgical wound dehiscence – 9 POD followed the primary operation.

Diagnosis

The diagnostic of postoperative peritonitis is based on the clinical signs and symptoms of patient.

Symptoms

Abdominal pain - usually generalized one - is the most frequently encountered complaint. Sometimes the pain may be not significantly intense due to the sedative and analgesic therapy, administered in the postoperative period. It is very difficult to be distinguished from the usual – related to the operative injury on the tissues – postoperative pain and avoiding of movement due to the pain, in the presence of other ascertainment, which define the condition as peritonitis.

The gradual increase of the abdominal swelling is the next most important finding. It results in difficulties in breathing, and reduces the mobility upon respiration of the abdominal wall. The abdominal ballooning requires distinguishing from paralytic or mechanical ileus, caused by other factors. However, because peritonitis itself causes progressive paralytic ileus, the following has to be noted: the increasing secretion from the nasogastric tube, nausea, vomiting (sometimes despite the tube and what takes place around it), non-recovery or de novo stop in the flatus and defecation or watery foul-smelling diarrheal defecations with pathological components mixed in the faeces.

High grade of fever with chills are a sign of infection in the organism. Thus, the newly occurred – in the postoperative period (after laparotomy) – febricity always indicates infectious complication as one of the possibilities for development of postoperative peritonitis.

Dehiscence of the surgical wound, intestinal, biliary, or purulent secretion from it, as well as from the drainages, are signs indicating serious failures, related to the initial operation.

Increased body temperature, tachycardia, and tachypnea with hypotension suggest a syndrome of systemic inflammatory reaction and – in patient after laparotomy performed – they are an indication for possible development of peritonitis.

Poor nutrition, paleness, and dehydration can be factors, which contribute to the development of peritonitis due to weakened immunological response and/or to be consequence from development of septicemia.

Icterus, cyanosis, and edema can be indicators for worsening of the systemic inflammatory response – systemic inflammatory response syndrome (SIRS) towards development of multi organ development syndrome (MODS).

In the terminal stage, the acquirement Hippocratic facies is a characteristic, but, unfortunately, late sign.

Surgical Condition ("Status Hirurgicus")

Surgical Examination

Upon inspection – generalized swelling of abdomen with reduced mobility of abdominal wall upon respiration.

Upon palpation – the manifestation of generalized tenderness upon palpation with muscular defence to an extent of rigidity, and positive Blumberg's sign, are obvious proofs for peritonitis.

The surgical wound with characteristic pathological appearance – with purulent/biliary/small intestinal or feculent secretion, with dehiscence or similar secretion from the wound drains are explicit signs for already present postoperative peritonitis.

Upon percussion and auscultation – present free fluid in the abdomen, peristaltic sound that resembles splashing, or absence of peristaltic sounds, and noises, are usual ascertainment in finding of the complication.

Upon rectal digital examination, bloating of the anterior rectal wall can be found with tenderness and increased rectal temperature plus positive symptom of Lennander.

Laboratory Examinations

Worsening leukocytosis with leftward shift, increase of C-reactive protein, hypoproteinemia, and hypoalbuminemia are primary signs, followed by the characteristic hematological and biochemical constellation in development of SIRS-sepsis.

Radiological Examinations

Survey radiograph (often lateral radiograph) of abdomen can disclose obliteration of the retroperitoneal adipose view planes, and psoas shadow, which demonstrates peritoneal edema. The intestinal loops filled with gas, which have thickened, opaque walls, can be found upon development of paralytic ileus with edema of the intestinal walls.

Ultrasound examination can demonstrate free fluid in the abdomen with absence of intestinal peristalsis or thickening and swelling of peritoneum, omentum, or intestinal wall. The diagnostic aspiration of fluid under ultrasound control is a risk operation, but it has high accuracy and specificity.

CT and MRI have high diagnostic value but they are not applied routinely due to the difficult technical implementation, especially in the early postoperative period, and in patients with severe general condition and/or on mechanical ventilation, and also due to the high price.

ASSESSMENT OF SEVERITY AND PROGNOSIS

Diagnostics and Identification of Patients in High Risk

The rapid and accurate making of diagnosis cooperates for the earlier application of proper plan of treatment. The early clinical assessment is of essential significance for the making of diagnosis of complicated intraabdominal infections (cIAI). The clinical and laboratory examinations confirm the presence and degree of inflammatory reaction, while the imaging examinations (ultrasound and computed tomography) are a valuable addition to the clinical assessment. By means of prognostic scales (APACHE II, SOFA, qSOFA) patients with sepsis and high risk of development of complications and lethal outcome are identified, as well as the need for admission at Intensive Care Unit is determined.

The presence of some factors in patients with cIAI determine increased risk for development of organ failure, and respectively increased morbidity and mortality. Factors on the part of patient are: advanced age (reduced physiological reserves and limited response to stressors), existing comorbidity, immunosuppression, preceding administration of antibiotics, oncological disease, and poor physical status. Factors on the part of disease are: severity of disease at the time of admission, sepsis/septic shock, high score according to the assessment scales APACHE II, SOFA, delay of the surgical intervention (usually ≥ 24 hours), inability of control of the source of infection. Patients with several risk factors as for instance advanced age or severe intraabdominal infection with sepsis/septic shock, have exceptionally high risk of lethal outcome. Patients with "low" risk may become patients with "high" risk, if the "window of opportunities" is omitted in connection with diagnostics, resuscitation, and timely onset of treatment.

Prognostic Scales

In the clinical practice different models for scoring are used for assessment of severity of disease or for prognosis of the outcome of patients with sepsis. The most important tool for finding of inflammation, infection, and complications remains the criteria for SIRS: body temperature ≥ 38.0° or ≤ 36.0°; heart rate ≥ 90 beats per minute; respiratory rate ≥ 20 breaths per minute or carbon dioxide partial pressure ≤ 33 mm Hg; leukocytes ≥ 12 000 / mm3 or ≤ 4 000 / mm3 or ≥ 10% immature neutrophils [41]. The used prognostic scales in patients with cIAI are generally divided into two groups: scales for assessment of the severity of organ failure (Intensive Care Unit, ICU), and specific (surgical) scales for assessment of peritonitis.

The scales APACHE II (Acute Physiologic Assessment and Chronic Heart Evaluation II) or SAPS (Simplified Acute Physiology Score), which evaluate various organ systems for presence of dysfunction, while parameters from the first 24 hours of the stay of patient at ICU are used; they are also applicable in patients with peritonitis [42]. According to the scale APACHE II the severity of disease is determined as mild to moderately severe (< 15 score) or as severe (≥ 15 score). The SOFA

(Sequential [Sepsis-related] Organ Failure Assessment) scale allows the clinicians to monitor in dynamics the development of the pathological process in critically ill patients during the stay at the ICU by means of calculation of the number of affected organs and severity of their dysfunction by six organ systems (respiratory system, cardiovascular system, liver, kidneys, central nervous system, coagulation system) [43]. The organ dysfunction is considered as life-threatening, if the score by SOFA has increased with ≥ 2 points. Because the SOFA scale is not always accessible outside of Department of Anesthesia and Intensive Care (DAIC) (e.g., at emergency department or surgical department) as a tool for quick assessment and screening for sepsis, it is suggested the quick (q) SOFA scale, which includes three easy for assessment criteria: 1) change of consciousness (Glasgow Coma Scale < 15 score); 2) respiratory rate ≥ 22 breaths per minute; and 3) systolic blood pressure ≤ 100 mm Hg. Patients, who meet these criteria, have longer hospital stay, and increased risk of lethal outcome. The SOFA (at ICU) and qSOFA (at emergency department) scales identify patients with sepsis and determine the need for admission at ICU.

The score by the specific (surgical) scales for assessment of peritonitis is calculated a single time during surgery, and it frequently includes data from the intraoperative finding regarding the degree of contamination. The universal prognostic scales, which are independent from the etiology of peritonitis, are: P POSSUM (Physiological and Operative Severity Score for the enumeration of Mortality and morbidity), MPI (Mannheim Peritonitis Index), PIA (Peritonitis Index Altona) [44]. The MPI scale uses simple factors (grade of peritonitis, age, sex, presence of organ failure, presence of malignant disease, continuation of peritonitis of > 24 hours, origin of sepsis, type of exudate), and it is a reliable mean for assessment of the risk, and classification of patients with peritonitis. The surgical scales can be processed for specific diseases, as for example left-sided colonic PSS (Peritonitis Severity Score) [45], PULP Score [46], etc.

Another scale for assessment of cIAI is the scale WSES from the multicenter prospective study WISS [47]. The score by WSES/WISS, calculated at the time of admission of patient, includes factors for: 1) clinical state at the time of admission; 2) conditions of development of the disease; 3) delay in the control of source; and 4) risk factors, including age and immunosuppression. Score of more than 5.5 (range from 0 to ≥ 18) is the best predictor for mortality with high grade of sensitivity (89.2%) and specificity (83.5%).

These scales are unfortunately not sufficiently accurate to predict the individual prognosis for a particular patient.

One of the basic predictive parameters regarding mortality, as with the rest groups of peritonitis, is Mannheim Peritonitis Index (MPI), which was developed by Wacha and Linder [28] in the year 1983. It was developed based on retrospective analysis of data from 1 253 patients with peritonitis, among which 20 possible risk factors were considered. Only 8 of them turned out to have prognostic significance and were included in the MPI, i.e., they were classified by score for prognosis (Table 1).

Table 1. The Mannheim Peritonitis Index

Risk Factors	Points
Age > 50 years	5
Female sex	5
Organ failure *	7
Malignant process	4
Preoperative duration of peritonitis > 24 hours	4
Septic source outside of colon/rectum	4
Diffuse generalization of peritonitis	6
Exudate:	
serous	0
turbid, purulent	6
feculent	12

* Renal failure = creatinine > 177 mmol/L or urea > 167 mmol/L, or oliguria < 20 ml/hours; pulmonary failure = oxygen partial pressure < 50 mm Hg or carbon dioxide partial pressure > 50 mm Hg; intestinal obstruction/paresis > 24 hours or present mechanical ileus; hypo- or hyperdynamical shock.

The mortality increases proportionally depending on the result from MPI. Patients with score of 10 points have 15% risk of lethal outcome, while those with score of more than 26 points, are considered as having high risk for lethal outcome – 65%, despite the treatment administered/performed.

CAUSES FOR THE DELAY OF DIAGNOSIS MAKING OF POSTOPERATIVE PERITONITIS

It is always difficult some symptoms of the postoperative peritonitis to be differentiated from those of normal clinical manifestations after performed laparotomy. Abdominal pain usually cannot be distinguished from the so-called suture-line pain along the surgical wound or it can be absent, if a very good analgesia is achieved. Likewise, the swelling of abdomen, the absence of sounds - audible upon auscultation - from the intestines, nausea, vomiting, and absence of intestinal passage, etc., which presume paralytical ileus, can be present as normal postoperative course of behavior of the organism, especially in abdominal or pelvic operations of large dimensions, but also as a manifestation of the postoperative peritonitis. Likewise, the physical signs, related to pain upon palpation, rigidity, and muscular defence, can be insufficiently strongly manifested and informative, in contrast to the non-operated patients with peritonitis – primary or secondary. The febricity and tachycardia, which are among the most important characteristics of the postoperative peritonitis, can arise as a consequence of non-surgical inflammatory complication or due to even usual superficial thrombophlebitis at the site of maintenance of peripheral venous line.

Leukocytosis may also be present - usually in the normal course of early postoperative period. However, the de novo development of the clinical characteristics, repeated occurrence of pathological aberrations, after a certain period of improvement or absence of recovery of the parameters and functions after a period of time expected for this, suggests development of certain complications, the most serious of them being the postoperative peritonitis.

MANAGEMENT OF POSTOPERATIVE PERITONITIS

Principles

Intensive Care and Resuscitation

- overcoming of shock/hypovolemia and continuation of adequate tissue oxygenation
- antibacterial and antifungal therapy
- maintenance of the function of the already affected and potentially impaired organs and systems

It is known that in all cases of postoperative period, a certain degree of hypovolemia is observed due to the losses in the interstitial or "third" space. The velocity, in which the substitution is realized, depends on the degree of hypovolemia and physiological condition of patient. The effectiveness of infusion therapy is noted by normalization of pulse, blood pressure, and mental state. The placement of urinary catheter is of essential significance, because the recovery of excretion of urine is a reliable indicator for adequate fluid resuscitation. Invasive peripheral arterial blood-gas monitoring, and observation of central venous pressure via central venous line, are of particular importance in septic shock, advanced age or cardiac, pulmonary, or renal failure, in order to be ensured more accurate determination of the intravascular volume and cardiac output.

The oxygen therapy and – in more extreme circumstances – endotracheal intubation and mechanical ventilation were indicated in patients with sepsis.

Nasogastric decompression is applied in presence of ileus in order to be prevented pulmonary aspiration and to be reduced the pressure in the GIT.

The aggressive antibacterial therapy is determined in the beginning empirically, and after receiving of antibiotic susceptibility testing – according to the data of the latter. Postoperative intraabdominal infections in comparison with the tertiary peritonitis always requires surgical approach [29, 30, 31]. The greater part of patients are usually already involved by the antibiotic therapy, while the diagnosis is made, and the microbial etiologic factors tend to be multidrug resistant, including Enterococci (vancomycin-resistant Enterococci (VRE) as well), Gram-negative microorganisms (ESBL or AmpC or carbapenemase-producer), MRSA and Candida species. Thus, the choice of antibiotics in these cases must be influenced by the local epidemiology, and sensitivity of the isolates. Suitable means can be carbapenems, tigecycline, piperacilline/tazobactam or moxifloxacin depending on the microbial findings. Antimycotics are recommended in proved fungal infections.

Operative Treatment

An obligatory condition for success is the early, i.e., without delay, performing of the operative intervention for discontinuation of dissemination of microorganisms and adjuvants in the peritoneal cavity. All the rest measures are ineffective, if the operation does not liquidate the source of infection, and does not reduce drastically the numbers of microorganisms, which have already reached the peritoneal cavity and the amount of adjuvants, representing a prerequisite for maintenance of the infection, in order to be supported the reparative and immunological possibilities of the organism [33].

Tactics

Control of the Source of Infection
As a whole, the choice of procedure, as well as whether a certain type of "ectomy" or continuity/discontinuity resection will be performed – primary anastomosis (upon resection of the affected part – source of infection) with or without protective stoma, or exteriorization without performing of anastomosis, depends on the anatomical source of infection,

the degree of peritoneal inflammation, and the generalized septic response, as well as the premorbid reserves and comorbidity of patient.

The prevailing tendency is minimization of the risk from subsequent complication by means of avoiding of all intestinal suture lines in the presence of severe peritoneal inflammation.

Evacuation of Bacterial Inoculates, Pus, and Adjuvants (Aspiration, Debridement, Lavage)

Every non-vital or foreign material, including hemoglobin, in the peritoneal cavity potentiates the development of bacteria and causes serious infection. That is why all infectious fluids and adjuvants must be aspirated, while the hard particles must be removed [34, 35].

Three different approaches have been suggested:

Mechanical Cleaning

Cleaning of the peritoneal cavity with gauze pad, especially in connection with local peritonitis, was considered a method for reduction of dissemination of bacteria and local restriction of the process. However, it is currently distinct, that the bacterial contamination disseminates rapidly over the peritoneal cavity from the so called intraperitoneal circulation. [36].

Peritoneal Lavage

"Washing" of the peritoneal cavity with abundant amount of physiological saline, solution of antiseptics, or solution of antibiotics.

The problem is that the bacteria rapidly connect to the tissues, frequently by means of reaction between bacterial surface ligands and receptor cells. These bacteria are difficult to be removed by means of "slight" washing, although they can be removed by "pulsating jet irrigation" upon pressure of 70 psi [35, 36].

Irrigations with antiseptic solutions as povidone-iodium, chlorhexidine, etc., did not show the expected efficacy upon experimental and clinical studies [37].

Aggressive Debridement

Pedantic performing of debridement with opening of all cavities, removal of fibrin coating, and adjuvants. However, there exist objections regarding this method, the most serious of which is bleeding from injured surfaces as a result of deposition of hemoglobin and fibrin, which, as it is known, are powerful adjuvants that increase the risk of a subsequent infection [35].

- Decompression – treatment of abdominal compartment syndrome
- Treatment/avoiding of persisting or repeating infections

Uninterrupted/Fractionated Postoperative Peritoneal Lavage

Technique

It is performed by different ways – usually two installation catheters are placed in the subphrenic spaces and two evacuation drainage catheters of cavity lowest points of rectouterine pouch.

The term of the intermittent or uninterrupted irrigation usually varies from 1 to 5 days. Most authors add antibiotics or antiseptics in the fluid for performing of lavage. Frequently, however, by means of "canalization" of the fluid effective accomplishment of lavage of the whole peritoneal cavity is achieved.

Hallerback & Andersson [38] have evaluated continuous peritoneal irrigation upon treatment of purulent peritonitis in a prospective randomized study, and they have not found any clinical benefit from it.

Planned Relaparotomies or "Etappenlavage"

The planned relaparotomies, or "Etappenlavage," are defined as a series of planned several operative procedures, performed in an interval of 24 hours [33, 35] by means of re-exploration and sanative treatment in every procedure.

The abdomen can be closed temporarily with standard suture of the layers of abdominal wall (rarely) by means of use of provisory non-sealed sutures, zipper and Velcro-analogues (Figure 4).

The use of absorbing meshes reduces the abdominal pressure, prevents from prolapse, and provides a possibility for effective draining of the abdominal cavity; nevertheless, the development of necrosis with pressure ulcers of the intestinal wall, and formation of fistulas, is a possible complication [38]. Also, when this approach is used, patients must be subject to mechanical ventilation for a longer period of time after operation, which has its specific risks.

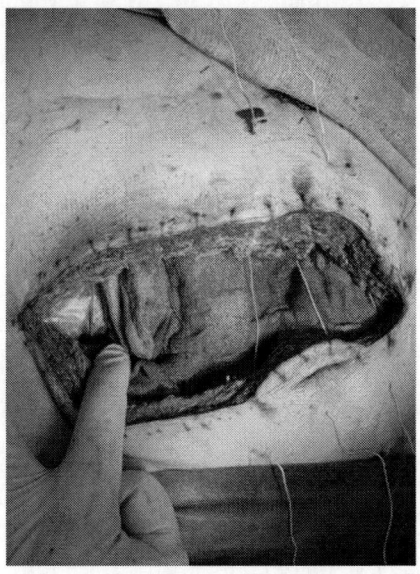

Figure 4 Temporary/incomplete closure of the abdominal wall in order - "Etappenlavage" in case of severe postoperative peritonitis.

Indications for Step-by-Step Closure of the Abdominal Cavity

- critical condition of patient having diffuse or total peritonitis with risk of development of multi organ dysfunction syndrome
- pronounced peritoneal edema, preventing abdominal closure without unnecessary pressure, upon intraabdominal pressure of > 15 mm Hg
- massive loss of abdominal wall
- impossible removing or controlling of the source of infection

- incomplete debridement of necrotic tissues
- insecurity of the vitality of intestinal sections
- uncontrolled bleeding (necessity of "packing")

Laparostomy (Open Abdominal Technique)

Open "packing" (with pads or a mesh) of the peritoneal cavity with delayed closure, recommended in patients with critical condition and with total purulent or feculent peritonitis (Figure 5). Thus, the whole abdominal cavity is treated with step-by-step (daily) revisioning of all sections, sanative treatment, and correction of drainage. Steinberg, 1979 [25] attempted this technique, and found dramatical improvement in the result. Duff & Moffat [39] confirmed the ascertainment and conclusion, that leaving the abdomen completely opened, facilitates as wide drainage as possible, thorough manipulation of wounds of abdominal wall, and is related with better recovery. The mortality rate is 34%. Anderson [40], however, did not find any advantage from preserving the abdomen open in patients with severe peritonitis. Counter to other authors, he reports of 60% mortality, compared to 33% in the control group, and increase of postoperative complications. As with "Ettapenlavage," in this technique patients need mechanical maintenance of respiration with average period with mechanical ventilation in the series of Duff and Moffat of 44 days.

A lot more is necessary to be done in this field with the purpose to be developed standards of management, which to be generally accepted.

The approach of Negative Pressure Wound Therapy has become widely used in contemporary surgical practice in the treatment of the septic abdomen as a complementary approach in the application of the laparostomy method. A special fenestrated cover foil is used, which is placed on the exposed area of the peritoneal cavity, protecting the peritoneal organs from lesions and allowing the exudate to the absorbent system. The latter consists of fine pored foam's flexible structure adapts to irregular wound contours (Figure 6).

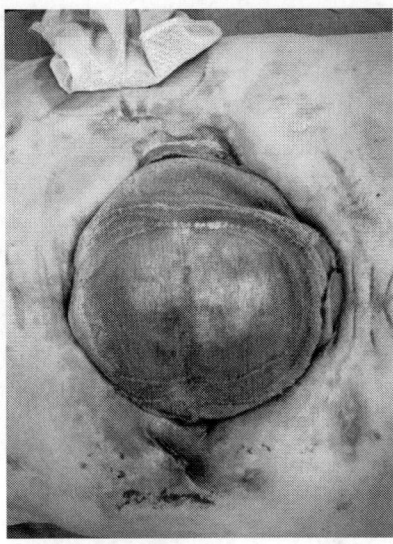

Figure 5. Laparostomy in case of feculent postoperative peritonitis.

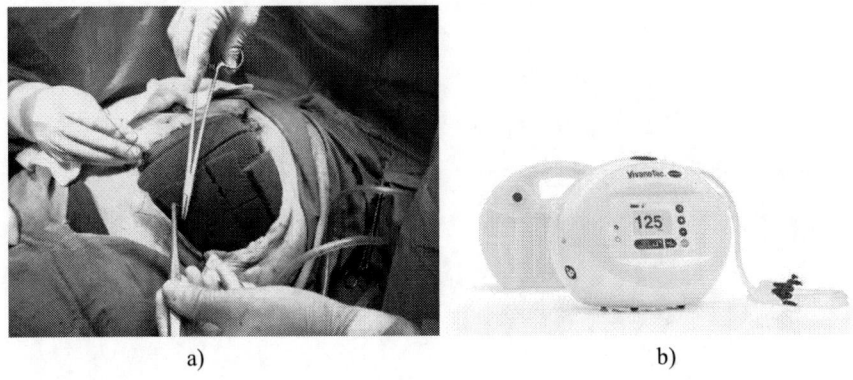

a)   b)

Figure 6. a) - Placing the microporous absorbent sponge above the barrier foil; b) negative pressure aspirator (*-adapted from Negative pressure wound therapy unit VivanoTec®).

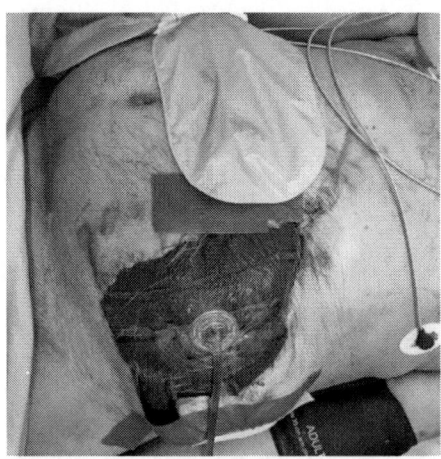

Figure 7. Adapted to the VacPack-system laparostomy.

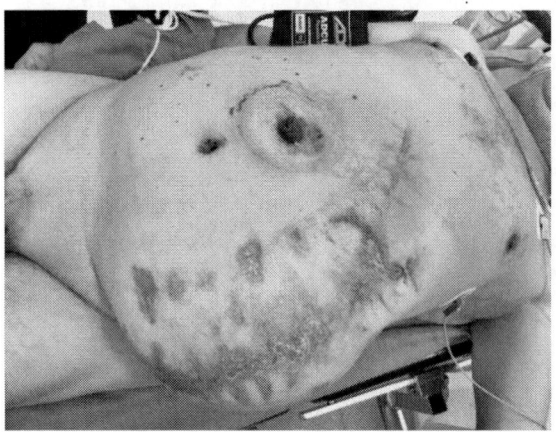

Figure 8. Definitive closed abdominal cavity after administration of VacPack-Laparostomy.

Due to the open-pored structure, the vacuum-pressure is distributed uniformly across the foam, which permits an efficient therapy. The sponge is covered with an adhesive sterile foil, which is attached to the skin around the laparostomy and the vacuum removes the exudate through a special adapter to the hose (Figure 7). Negative pressure is generated by various therapeutic modalities, subject to adjustment, by a special portable aspiration generator. The exudate is collected in a specially attached to the aspirator exudate canister, which contains solidifying gel packs and hydrophobic charcoal filter. Each canister is disposable, replaceable, sterile and individually packed with a capacity of 300 – 800 ml. The negative pressure therapy ensures the safe removal of peritoneal exudate and the promotion of tissue healing, stimulating cell growth and blood circulation in the affected tissues and organs; moreover, it provides a gradual reduction of pathological intra-abdominal hypertension and pulling together the two sides of the open abdominal wall which provides a subsequent definitive closure of the abdomen (Figure 8).

Intensive Care Aspects in the Treatment of Complicated Intra-Abdominal Infection

In the treatment of patients with complicated intraabdominal infections (cIAI) it is of first-rate significance, the conception, that the sepsis is an emergency condition and that the early identification, and the suitable immediate treatment in the first hours after its development, reduces the complications to a minimum and improves the outcome [48, 49]. The peritonitis is an absolute indication for extreme hospitalization.

The principles of treatment of patients with cIAI (sepsis, shock) include [50-52]:

1. Quick diagnostics and identification of patients with high risk;
2. Control of the source of infection (sepsis) / impairment (trauma) – liquidation of the source of peritonitis; evacuation of the exudate, sanative treatment, and drainage of the abdominal cavity;
3. Antibacterial therapy;
4. Intensive care for recovery of the function of vital organs and systems.

Intensive Preoperative Preparation

The intensive preoperative preparation of patient with cIAI begins immediately after the diagnosis making, continues briefly (2 to 6 hours), and includes:

1. Infusion therapy with the use of a protocol of early goal-directed therapy (EGDT), and criteria for adequacy: central venous pressure – 8-12 mm Hg; mean arterial pressure $\geq$ 65 mm Hg; excretion of urine > 0.5 ml/kg/h; central venous oxygen saturation > 70%. It usually begins with administration of crystalloids (Ringer lactate solution or physiological saline). The discussions, regarding the risk/benefit of the use of colloids in patients with sepsis, continue. In persistence of hypotension and hypoperfusion vasopressors are to be added without delay (noradrenaline, vasopressin, dopamine), and corticosteroids (upon refractory septic shock – hydrocortisone 200-300 mg/daily or equivalent bolus for a period of not less than 100 hours). Frequent reassessment of the hemodynamical state is recommended, placement of catheter of a central vein in order to be monitored the infusion therapy and to be administered vasoactive agents. The level of lactate in blood is monitored and upon values of more than 2 mmol/l (as a marker for tissue perfusion) the examination is repeated within 2-4 hours. Hemotransfusion (in levels of hemoglobin of less than 70 g/l - in adults upon absence of conditions as myocardial ischemia, severe hypoxemia, or acute hemorrhage) is also performed as needed.

2. Early (during the first hour from the moment of patient's admission at the inpatient unit) parenteral (intravenous) administration of empirical antibacterial broad-spectrum therapy in adequate start doses as monotherapy or in combination with metronidazole. Regimens of antimicrobial preparations have to be used with activity against the typical Gram-negative Enterobacteriaceae, Gram-positive cocci, and obligate anaerobes, which participate in these infections. The recommended antibiotics for monotherapy and regimens for administration are: piperacillin/tazobactam – 4.5 g once every 6 hours i.v. slow jet administration (for 3-5 minutes) or drip infusion (for not less than 20-30 minutes); imipenem/cilastatin (1.0 g once every 8 hours); meropenem (1.0 g once every 8 hours); doripenem (0.5 g once every 8 hours); ertapenem – 1.0 g once daily i.v. administration for 30 minutes; tigecycline – 100 mg i.v. loading dose, followed by 50 mg once every 12 hours; moxifloxacin – 400 mg once daily i.v. administration for 60 minutes. If the cause of peritonitis is destruction of appendix, colon, or terminal ileum,

metronidazole is also added. The cephalosporins (cefepime in a dose of 1.0-2.0 g twice daily i.v., or cephalosporin of third generation in a dose 1.0-2.0 g twice daily) are used in combination with metronidazole 0.5 g three times daily i.v. administration. Aztreonam – 1.0-2.0 g three times daily i.v. administration plus metronidazole 0.5 g three times daily i.v. administration. Upon disturbance of renal function, the doses are corrected according to the creatinine clearance. When micotic infection is suspected (or such is proved), a suitable antimicotic is added to the therapy. If Candida albicans is isolated, a mean of choice is fluconazole, while in the other types of Candida (C. krusei, C. glabrata) the use of voriconazole, caspofungin, and amphotericin B is purposeful.

The collecting of suitable biological materials (including blood cultures; always at least two sets of aerobes and anaerobes) for microbiological examination must precede the initiation of antibiotic therapy in order to be optimized the identification of pathogens.

3. Placement of nasogastric tube (NGT) for evacuation of gastric content.

4. Placement of urethral catheter for monitoring of the hourly excretion of urine.

5. Hygiene preparation in the field of operative intervention.

Control of the Source of Infection

In order to be achieved elimination of the source of infection and control of the continuous contamination, surgical treatment is performed. The main goal of treatment in extreme surgery is saving of the life of patient and the supposed dimensions of operative intervention must be consistent with functional abilities of patients with cIAI and septic shock.

The surgical sanative treatment in cIAI must be realized as quick as possible after diagnosis making and must be maximally adequate, because any delay or inadequately performed surgical intervention may influence negatively the outcome of disease [53, 54]. The time for performing of the operation is an independent predictor for clinical failure in patient with cIAI. There are two contradictory trends of activity in the literature until the moment of radical sanative treatment of the source. According to one of them – the surgical sanative treatment must be performed in maximally brief periods of time with the purpose of reduction of bacterial loading before the progressing worsening of the condition of patient with development of refractory septic shock, while according to the other one – first-rate task is the primary stabilization of the hemodynamic and physiological state of patient, and subsequent operation [55].

In septic shock, the achievement of complete resuscitation is impossible before discontinuation of the distribution of infectious process, and sometimes the operation can be a part of the complex of resuscitation measures. In most patients with cIAI operative treatment is undertaken after stabilization of the general condition and correction of the metabolic disturbances during a reasonable time interval up to the intervention. Upon rapid worsening of the disease (intraabdominal hypertension, necrotizing fasciitis), however the operative intervention is to be realized within < 1-2 hours after making of the diagnosis in parallel with the administered intensive therapy. In the cases of pancreatic necrosis, surgical treatment is undertaken after demarking of the infectious process and delineation of the inflammation. However, the moment of emergency for performing of the surgical intervention is a problematic, complex decision, and is determined individually for every particular patient in the context of his/her disease [56-58].

The surgical intervention (extensive median laparotomy or laparoscopy) remains the most purposeful therapeutic strategy for treatment of cIAI, it is performed in the setting of general anesthesia, and has for its aim finding and liquidation of the source of peritonitis (e.g., resection or suture of perforated organ, removal of infected organ), evacuation of exudate, sanative treatment, and rational draining of abdominal cavity, as well as draining of intestines, which – in the forms of peritonitis with dissemination – are in the state of paresis. Depending on the local finding, a variant for the primary operation is chosen (primary closure of abdominal cavity or laparostomy), and determination of further tactics in the management of patient (e.g., elective or on demand relaparotomies) [50, 52].

The ending of operation with laparostomy is indicated in patients in unstable condition with sepsis; this relieves the subsequent control of the condition of abdominal cavity and prevents the development of the state of intraabdominal hypertension (IAH) and abdominal compartment syndrome (ACS) [50, 59, 60]. The temporary closure of abdominal cavity creates serious problems for the intensive care physicians, related to electrolyte disturbances, hypovolemia, nutritional insufficiency, formation of intestinal fistulas, and loss of abdominal wall.

Planned relaparotomy is used upon inability for single-moment removal or reliable delineation of the source of peritonitis with complete sanative treatment of abdominal cavity; presence of IAH; suspicion for the vitality of intestines and consistency of intestinal anastomoses; formed multiple abscesses between the folds; need to be performed delayed intraabdominal anastomoses. Upon need for relaparotomy in high-risk patients with severe peritonitis (MPI < 20 score; APACHE II < 14 score), in which an adequate control over the focus of infection is achieved during the first operation – on demand relaparotomy is preferably [52]. As a rule the on demand relaparotomy is performed in connection with worsening of the clinical condition of patient or upon absence of improvement, and it is an effective measure for liquidation of permanent or repeated infecting of the abdominal cavity.

After re-exploration – if the condition of patient allows it – early and definitive closure of the abdominal cavity is considered, with the aim of reduction of complications, related with the open abdomen (e.g., enteroatmospheric fistulas, retraction of the fascia, development of incisional hernias) [61, 62]. The temporary closure of abdominal cavity with the use of negative pressure (negative pressure therapy, NPT) can be helpful for shortening of the time until the definitive closure of abdominal cavity. The continuous administration of NPT may increase the risk for formation of intestinal fistulas.

A material for microbiological examination is always collected intraoperatively, including after each reoperation. The material collected in aseptic setting from abdominal cavity (usually at least 1-2 ml fluid or tissue) is placed in a container with transport environment and is transported as quickly as possible at the microbiological laboratory, in order to be avoided compromise of samples. In the laboratory, the intraperitoneal specimen is immediately examined under a microscope with Gram staining, examination for aerobes and anaerobes with cultures, and generation of antibiotic susceptibility testing. Collecting of samples with a pad is not recommended!

Antibacterial Therapy

The antibacterial therapy is an additional method to the surgical treatment of cIAI [62]. On absence of control over the focus of infection, it is a basic method for treatment of infection.

According to the etiology, cIAI are usually polymicrobial. In connection with community-acquired infection, the spectrum of pathogens is sufficiently predictable and limited to representatives of Enterobacteriaceae (mainly Escherichia coli and Klebsiella spp.), viridans group streptococci, and anaerobes (especially Bacteroides fragilis). Upon nosocomial essence of the peritonitis and intraabdominal sepsis, regardless of the leading role of the above-mentioned etiological agents, their spectrum is less predictable and extended at the expense of Gram-negative non-fermenting bacteria (Pseudomonas spp., Acinetobacter spp.), etc. The most frequently isolated Gram-positive pathogens are Enterococcus spp.

The primary antibiotic therapy is empirical, because data from the microbiological examination (with cultures and regarding sensitivity), suitable for more detailed analysis, are available only after $\geq$ 24 hours. The principles of empirical antibiotic therapy are based on the source of infection and the most probable pathogenic etiological agent. The etiology of cIAI varies depending on the site of source with dissemination of Gram-positive pathogens, and Candida spp. in the upper sections of gastrointestinal tract (GIT) and progressive increase of the anaerobes and Gram-negative pathogens in the lower sections of GIT. When the choice of empirical antibiotic therapy is to be done, the local tendency for antibiotic resistance has to be considered.

During the last few years, the distribution of cIAI - caused by multi-resistant microorganisms - dramatically increased. In the nosocomial infections can be encountered Gram-positive, as well as Gram-negative multi-resistant pathogens, as MRSA (methicillin-resistant Staphylococcus aureus), VRE (vancomycin-resistant enterococci) and ESBL (extended-spectrum beta lactamases) producing Enterobacteriaceae, as well as CRE (carbapenem-resistant Enterobacteriaceae), multi-resistant Pseudomonas aeruginosa and Acinetobacter spp. The most important factors for presence of multi-resistant pathogens in cIAI is the preceding antibiotic therapy, hospitalization for more than one week, preceding therapy with corticosteroids, organ transplantation, initial lung or liver disease, and reoperations. There are currently reports for resistant causative agents upon infections with community-acquired origin as well, which preconditions the need for thorough analysis of every clinical case for finding of risk factors in the medical history [63].

The adequate antibacterial therapy must include: administration of loading dose of the preparation upon presence of indications, especially in patients in critical condition; permanent or extended infusion of beta-lactamase antibiotics; monitoring of the concentration of medicines (peritoneal distribution). In peritonitis and abdominal sepsis, caused by nosocomial pathogen, as preparations of choice there is recommendation for considering of meropenem, imipenem, doripenem, and also inhibitor-protected anti-Pseudomonas beta-lactams (cefoperazone/sulbactam, piperacillin/tazobactam) [63, 64]. The regimen of administration of the antibiotic therapy is to be observed again once daily, because the pathophysiological changes can have significant influence on the biological availability of the medicines.

The results from the microbiological examination have major significance for the choice of therapeutic strategy on every patient and specifically in the adaptation of the target antibiotic treatment. In connection with acquiring of the results for the causative agents of cIAI and their sensitivity, de-escalation, change, or discontinuation of the antibiotic therapy are considered. When adequate surgical control - of the focus of infection in cIAI – is exerted, brief (3-5 days) courses of antibiotic therapy are recommended.

The criteria for effectiveness of the antibiotic therapy in peritonitis and abdominal sepsis are the positive dynamics of the symptoms of IAI, decrease of body temperature, reduction of intoxication, and degree of systemic inflammatory response. Upon persistent signs of peritonitis or signs of infection after five-day antibiotic therapy, it is necessary to be performed diagnostic searching on the base of clinical assessment, clinical and laboratory (including c-reactive protein, and procalcitonin), and imaging examinations for finding of residual infection, resistant microorganisms, and other possible factors for therapy failure, and not simply continuation or extension of the antimicrobial therapy [50]. The data from cultures, collected from abdominal drains, placed more than 48 hours ago, are to be interpreted attentively, because biofilm is formed and colonization occurs. For this reason, the routine collecting of materials for microbiological examination of such drains is not recommended.

When the modern antimicotial therapy is considered in patients with cIAI, treated at Intensive Care Units, the following has to be considered: 1) the quick identification of the particular pathogens, which caused IAI, shortens the period of empirical broad-spectrum antimicrobial therapy; 2) at every Intensive Care Unit with surgical patients, a control has to be realized on the use of antibiotics in order to be avoided adverse drug reactions (as renal and/or hepatic failure), avoiding of bacterial resistance; and 3) differentiation between infection and colonization.

The absence of control on the source of infection and adequacy of antibacterial therapy are the only modified risk factors for the mortality in patients with cIAI, hospitalized at ICU. In the setting of increasing resistance, data are found that the significance of control on the focus of infection replaces the influence of the antibiotic therapy [65]. The development and application in the clinical practice of protocols for treatment of cIAI based on the local epidemiology with the profile of resistance, and the local administration of antimicrobial agents will improve the quality of care in patients with cIAI. Such local directions must be established by a multidisciplinary team, including a surgeon, infectious disease specialist, hospital microbiologist, and intensive care physician, and are to reflect the local resources and standards for care.

Postoperative Intensive Care Continues at ICU, and Includes [64]

1. Continuation of the empirical antibacterial therapy with broad-spectrum antibiotic according to the chosen regimen of initial therapy. After identification of the pathogen(s) and establishment of the sensitivity, empirical antibiotic therapy (48-72 hours from the beginning) can change or the spectrum of activity can narrow.
2. Antimycotic therapy in patients with proved causative agent for fungal infection or risk for development of secondary fungal infection: fluconazole 400 mg once daily with slow i.v. administration for 60 minutes, followed by 200 mg daily; or caspofungin 70 mg once daily with slow i.v. administration for 60 minutes, followed by 50 mg daily; or micafungin 100 mg once daily with slow i.v. administration for 60 minutes.
3. Effective infusion therapy – crystalloids, colloids, vasopressors (noradrenaline, vasopressin [up to 0.03 U/min], dopamine – preparations and doses by indications according to data from monitoring), corticosteroids (upon refractory septic shock of 200-300 mg daily hydrocortisone or equivalent), albumin; precise monitoring (central venous pressure – 8-12 mm Hg; mean arterial pressure $\geq$ 65 mm Hg; excretion of urine > 0.5 ml/kg/h; central venous oxygen saturation > 70%) for avoiding of loading with fluids, which can result in pulmonary edema, intestinal edema, and increase of the intraabdominal pressure and development of abdominal compartment syndrome (ACS).
4. Mechanical ventilation (MV) in the presence of data of respiratory failure. The recommended strategy for ventilator maintenance in patients with acute respiratory distress syndrome (ARDS) include ventilation in low volumes (6 ml/kg) and limited pressure in the respiratory tract (plateau pressure of $\leq$ 30 cm H_2O) with application of positive end-expiratory pressure (PEEP) for preventing of expiratory collapse of the alveoli and improvement of oxygenation. The bed has to be in position of raised head at 30-45°.

5. Sedation for adaptation to MV is recommended to be performed as briefly as possible with interruptions in the day hours.
6. Intra- and extracorporeal detoxification – forced excretion of urine, plasmapheresis, hemodiafiltration. The main reason for the use of extracorporeal cleaning of blood in patients with cIAI, and septic shock, is removal of inflammatory cytokines and modulation of the immune response.
7. Adequate coping with pain – opioids, non-opioid analgesics, and continuous epidural analgesia. The pain is an important factor for postoperative complications (e.g., lung complications), and extended inpatient stay.
8. Prophylaxis of the venous thromboembolism with low molecular weight heparin (LMWH) or standard heparin on absence of contraindications for the use of these agents. The use of LMWH is recommended on absence of contraindications, because the use of standard heparin is related to increased frequency of heparin-induced thrombocytopenia (HIT). The combination of pharmacological agents and intermittent pneumatic compression is recommended.
9. Prophylaxis and treatment of coagulopathies with monitoring of control coagulogram.
10. Correction of aqueous-electrolyte disturbances.
11. Correction of hypo- and dysproteinemia.
12. Hemotransfusion upon septic anemia (recommended level of hemoglobin – not less than 90 g/l).
13. Stimulation of the function of intestines: enema, anticholinesterase preparations (e.g., neostigmine, galantamine), gastrokinetics (e.g., metoclopramide), enteral nutrition.
14. Nutritional maintenance, including trophic/hypocaloric nutrition (of up to 500 kcal/daily, or 10 to 20 kcal/hourly, or 70% of the caloric targets) and/or early enteral nutrition (by means of feeding tube) with increase of the volume in compliance with the tolerance. Routine monitoring of the volume of residual gastric content is

necessary, especially in patients with increased risk from aspiration.
15. Glycemic control (target at blood glucose level < 10 mmol/l). Initiation of therapy with insulin upon two consecutive measurements of blood glucose ≥ 10 mmol/l.
16. Stress ulcer prophylaxis of GIT or with proton pump inhibitors (PPIs) or H2 blockers, enteral nutrition.
17. Rehabilitation – accelerated achievement by patient of ability to keep balance in vertical position.

Routine daily care for patients with cIAI at ICU must be based on the main aspects in the modern intensive care of critically ill patients, described as FAST-HUG (Feeding, Analgesia, Sedation, Thromboembolic prophylaxis, Head-of-bed elevation, stress Ulcer prevention, Glucose control) [66, 67]. For the successful treatment of patients with cIAI the efforts of different specialists must be united in one team.

COMPLICATIONS FROM POSTOPERATIVE PERITONITIS

The complications can be divided into the following groups:

1. Intraabdominal complications – abscesses, enterocutaneous fistulas, stress-ulcer of GIT, abdominal compartment syndrome, adhesive ileus, insufficiency of intestinal anastomoses.
2. Complications from the anterior abdominal wall and retroperitoneum – phlegmon, purulent surgical would, eventration.
3. Extraabdominal complications – deep venous thrombosis, pulmonary thromboembolism, pneumonia, pleurisy, mediastinitis, abdominal compartment syndrome.

Intraabdominal Hypertension – Abdomen Compartment Syndrome

The intraabdominal pressure (IAP) is submitted to the hydrostatic laws and is defined by the state of intraabdominal organs and structures, which determine the borders of abdominal cavity (spine, pelvis, and costal arch – non-elastic structures; diaphragm and abdominal wall – elastic structures). Likewise every other anatomical compartment (as cranial cavity, pericardial space, etc.), the abdominal cavity has limited capacity to extent and upon insufficiency between its volumetric capacity and volume of the content, the pressure in this closed limited space may increase without control.

In the severe forms of peritonitis with development of abdominal sepsis not infrequently is observed increase of IAP, which may result in state of permanent or repeating pathological increase of IAP to more than 12 mm Hg, known as intraabdominal hypertension (IAH). IAH results in disturbance of blood circulation, hypoperfusion and ischemia of the organs and tissues in the abdominal cavity with subsequent dysfunction (abdominal compartment syndrome). ACS is a complex of symptoms, which develops as a result of continuous increase of IAP to more than 20 mm Hg, and is characterized with severe disturbances of the systemic perfusion and development of multiple organ dysfunction syndrome (MODS). The causes for occurrence of intraabdominal hypertension (IAH) are the presence of fluid in the abdominal cavity (e.g., exudate, blood), paresis of intestines and edema of internal organs, as well as the massive infusion/transfusion therapy in resuscitation measures, closure of surgical wound on excessive strain on the abdominal wall tissues, the early postoperative period. IAH has negative influence on the function of actually all organs and systems in the organism (cardiorespiratory, gastrointestinal, urinary, and central nervous system) and is related to the complicated course of disease, postoperative complications, and high postoperative mortality [68].

The clinical signs and symptoms, and the physical assessment of abdominal state, are not sufficiently exact for diagnosis specification of IAH/ACS. In the year 2007, based on a consensus, the World Society of the Abdominal Compartment Syndrome (WSACS) published Recommendations for Measurement of IAP and Treatment of IAH/ACS (updated in 2013) [69]. The method of choice and golden standard for diagnostics of ACS is the measurement of IAP in urinary bladder. This small invasive technique does not require complex equipment, allows easy, accurate and quick measurement of IAP coupled with low prime cost. ACS is diagnosed upon values of less than 20 mm Hg in combination with failure of more than one organ. IAP must be monitored in all patients with cIAI, for which it is considered that there is an increased risk (two or more risk factors) for significant increase of IAP. In these patients, IAP is measured at least 4-6 times daily, or more frequently in patients with unstable hemodynamic or rapid deteriorating organ function. Upon stabilization of the condition, IAP is measured once per 24-48 hours.

The most effective treatment of IAH and ACS is the prophylaxis or early diagnostics (which is more realistic). Patients with IAH/ACS must be monitored in dynamics for: oliguria, increased peak inspiratory pressures in the respiratory tract/reduction of respiratory volume/hypoxemia/ hypercapnia, hypotension and reduction of the cardiac volume per minute, bleeding from the gastrointestinal tract (GIT), reduced circulation of the distal parts of limbs, increased intravesical pressure. Because all parameters are interrelated and influence one another, for the proper interpretation of parameters, and, respectively, for undertaking of proper therapy, it is necessary the values to be considered in the context of the overall constellation of clinical signs and symptoms. Upon IAH with measurement of IAP of 16-20 mm Hg, the standards of treatment include permanent monitoring of IAP, of the functions of vital organs and administration of intensive conservative measures, including: 1) MV – protective lung ventilation with small respiratory volumes (6 mL/kg) with the purpose of preventing of barotrauma and ventilator-induced lung injury (VILI); 2) adequate infusion therapy – strict fluid balance (in order to be avoided exceeding positive balance); removal of hypovolemia with crystalloid and colloid solutions before the decompressive laparotomy; 3) gastrokinetics and stimulation of intestinal peristalsis with neostigmine; 4) decompression of GIT (nasogastric tube, gas tube in rectum); 5) inotropic agents and vasopressors – individualized approach; 6) renal replacement therapy (hemodialysis), in the presence of indications; 7) sedation, analgesia, muscular relaxation (synchronization with MV, reduction of strain on the abdominal musculature upon pain and psychomotor agitation); 8) position of the body – position reverse Trendelenburg is a compromise between raised head at 30° (for prophylaxis of aspiration syndrome related to mechanical ventilation) or at 20° (maximally acceptable raising of head upon IAH) [70, 71].

In the presence of absence of efficiency of the conservative treatment and impending ACS, laparotomy for abdominal decompression has to be performed [72, 73]. The surgical decompression of abdominal cavity is the only effective method for treatment of ACS. Upon increase of IAP of more than 35 mm Hg, the emergency surgical intervention has the characteristics of resuscitation, because IAH for only several hours can lead to rapidly progressing organ dysfunction and lethal outcome of patient. The decompressive laparotomy results in immediate reduction of IAP and improvement of organ function, but at the same time it may be accompanied by a number of complications, as acute heart failure (due to abrupt reduction of IAP, and overall peripheral vascular resistance and existing hypovolemia), thromboembolism and even cardiac arrest as a result of reperfusion, and great amounts of not completely oxidized substrates, and intermediate metabolic products, reaching the blood flow. The mortality reaches up to 50%. After performing of decompressive laparotomy, and on existing probability for worsening of ACS, the question for closure of abdominal cavity is solved [60]. Temporary plastic surgery is often performed with the use of special mesh-like implants (cloths) (Marlex, Prolene, Vypro, and analogous ones) without decrease of the volume of abdominal cavity. Some authors leave the abdomen open (laparostomy) with gradual liquidation of the abdominal wall defect according to the degree of solution of ACS and normalization of IAP. The longer is the period of time, in which patient remains with laparostomy, the higher is the morbidity.

Enterocutaneous Fistulas

The enterocutaneous fistula (ECF) is a complex and multiform pathology. It represents a pathological connection between gastrointestinal tract (GIT) and skin.

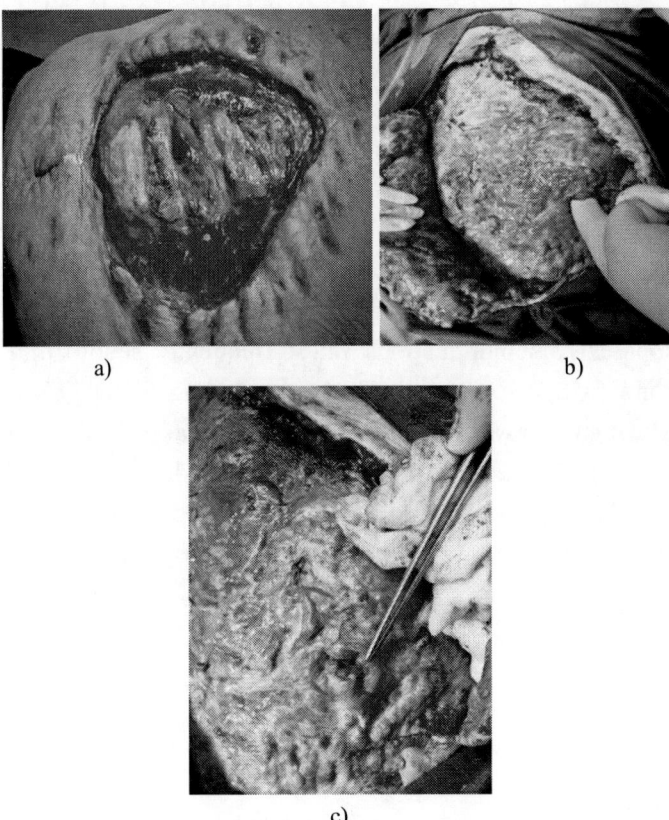

Figure 9. a,b,c Enterocutaneous fistula in "frozen abdomen."

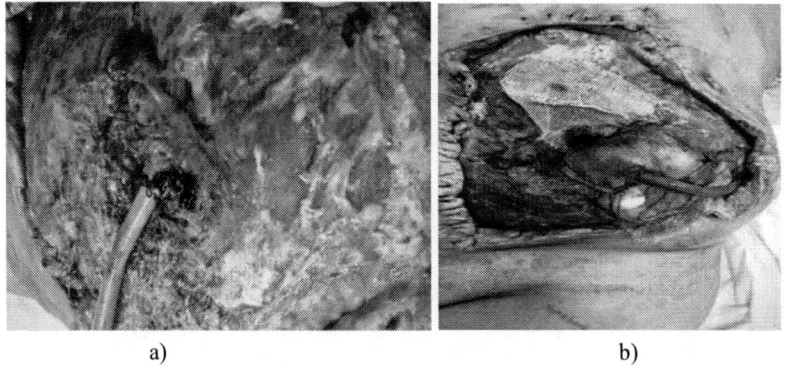

Figure 10. a, b "Tubage"-drainage of enterocutaneous fistula.

It most often occurs during inadequate or unsuccessful treatment with the laparostomy method, which results in the formation of massive planar adhesions between all intraperitoneal structures with complete obliteration of the peritoneal cavity with impaired peristaltic function of all intestinal segments, the so-called "frozen abdomen" (Figure 9). ECF causes complex disturbances in the homeostasis (dehydration, dyselectrolytemia, malnutrition, intoxication), and microcirculation, and is related to high risk for development of complications (most frequently septic), multisystem organ failure (MSOF), and lethal outcome (up to 85%) [74-77]. When intestinal content appears on the abdominal wall/surgical wound, the diagnosis making does not present particular difficulties. ECF is an exceptional challenge for treatment and requires coordinated care by the multidisciplinary team (surgeon, anesthesiologist, radiologist, gastroenterologist, and microbiologist) [78, 79] (Figure 10).

CLINICAL ISSUES

Secretion in GIT

Depending on the position of ECF, the volume and electrolyte composition of the lost intestinal content are different. The higher (more proximal) is situated the ECF, the more significant are the occurring pathophysiological disturbances in the organism: loss of intestinal content (averagely 1 600 ml/daily), enzymes (salivary amylase, gastric pepsin, powerful pancreatic proteolytic enzymes), electrolytes (sodium, potassium, magnesium, and chloride), and essential nutrients (Table 2). All of them cause dehydration, hypovolemia, changes in the rheological qualities of blood (increase of viscosity) with disturbances in the microcirculation, metabolic disturbances, reduction of glomerular filtration and excretion of urine, development of dysproteinemia with hypoalbuminemia, multisystem organ failure (MSOF).

Table 2. Daily secretion and composition of gastrointestinal secretions*

	Volume**	Na+	K+	Cl-	HCO3-	H-	pH
Saliva	1 500 (500-2 000)	10	26	10	30	0	6.0-7.0
Stomach	1 500 (100-4 000)	60	10	130	0	70-100	1.0-3.5
Duodenum (Brunner`s glands)	~200 (100-2 000)	140	5	80	0	0	8.0-8.9
Ileum	3 000 (100-9 000)	140	5	104	30	0	7.5-8.0
Pancreas	800 (100-800)	140	5	75	115	0	8.0-8.3
Bile	800 (50-800)	145	5	100	35	0	7.8
Colon	200	60	30	40	0	0	7.5-8.0

Adapted from: Gomella LG, Lefor AT. Surgery on Call. Norwalk, CT: Appleton-Lange; 1990.
* All electrolytes are presented in mEq/L.
** mL/day; the range of daily amount of secretion is presented in parentheses.

When septic complications (peritonitis, wound infection, etc.) are concomitant, the described disturbances are still more expressed and additionally worsen the course of disease. The changes in the aqueous-electrolyte and nutritional condition in case of ECF, located in the distal section of small intestine, are less expressed, and in most of large intestinal ECF, they are rarely observed. The high productive ECG ($\geq$ 500 ml/daily) are usually associated with issues related to the balance of fluids, decreased capacity of absorption for nutrients, as well as with poor prognosis [76, 80]. The main problems in large intestinal ECF are related to purulent septic processes in the surrounding tissues and abdominal cavity.

Malnutrition

Most patients with ECF (55-90%) have severe malnutrition (BMI < 20), which occurred acutely as a result of increased losses of nutrients through ECF, insufficient (limited) intake and disturbed intestinal absorption of nutrients, as well as of increased energy needs, related to the sepsis, and catabolic condition. The malnutrition in these patients is related to increased morbidity and mortality [76-78].

Skin Impairment

The secretions of ECF contain a number of proteolytic enzymes and bile salts, which can cause serious impairment of skin and surrounding tissues, causing inflammation, ulceration and possible infection. That is why the decrease of secretion from GIT and the early identification of the short bowel syndrome is an essential part of the treatment of patients with ECF and is of important significance for better results [76, 78, 79].

Therapy

The therapy of patients with ECF is still a difficult and unsolved problem. The most complex and difficult for treatment are the highly productive ($\geq$ 500 ml/daily), and multiple ECF, formed against the background of peritonitis. The irregular tactics of treatment not infrequently results in mistakes, additional new complications, relapses of ECF, and lethal outcome.

Initial resuscitation and stabilization	
Fluid replacement - rehydration	Electrolyte replacement therapy

⇓⇓⇓⇓⇓

Control of sepsis	
Antibacterial therapy	Infection source control

⇓⇓⇓⇓⇓

Nutrition	
Enteral nutrition	Parenteral nutrition

⇓⇓⇓⇓⇓

Control of fistula output	
Antisecretory agents	Wound/skin care
Antimotility agents	

⇓⇓⇓⇓⇓

Surgery	
Detailed plan of type of surgery	Timing of surgery

Figure 11. Treatment approach for patients with ECF.

The therapeutic strategies are diverse and include both conservative and surgical treatment. The generally accepted at present standards for treatment of patients with ECF are based on cohort of series and opinion of experts [75-77, 81-83]. The priorities of therapeutic measures are: 1) treatment of sepsis; 2) optimization of nutritional state; 3) wound care; 4) establishing of the anatomy of fistule; 5) developing of a plan for treatment with determination of the type of surgical intervention and suitable moment for its performing (Figure 11).

Conservative Therapy for Initial Stabilization

The initial stabilization of patients' condition is achieved by means of conservative treatment: correction of the aqueous electrolyte disorders (infusion therapy for rehydration and supplementation of electrolytes); treatment of purulent septic conditions (antibiotics, surgical treatment); nutritional maintenance (balanced parenteral and/or enteral nutrition); reduction or discontinuation of the losses through ECF (with pharmacological agents as H2 blockers, proton pump inhibitors, sandostatin); care of skin around ECF (creams, sprays). The treatment of patients who have sepsis and septic shock is performed according to the generally accepted instructions and recommendations, beginning with the early purposeful therapy (central venous pressure of 8-12 mm Hg, mean arterial pressure ≥ 65 mm Hg, excretion of urine ≥ 0.5 ml/kg/hour, and oxygen saturation of mixed venous blood ≥ 65%) [84].

After collecting of suitable samples for microbiological examination (blood culture, intraabdominal fluid/abscess, etc.) without delay empirical antimicrobial therapy with broad-spectrum antibiotics is initiated – meropenem, imipenem, cilastatin, piperacillin-tazobactam as monotherapy, or ceftriaxone/cefoperazone-sulbactam in combination with metronidazole. The antimycotics are administered in patients with proved fungal etiological agent or in patients with risk for development of secondary fungal infection [85]. Upon presence of intraabdominal infection, surgical sanative treatment is obligatory.

The nutritional maintenance improves and sustains the nutritive state of patient and enables achievement of as good as possible surgical result after recovery of ECF [83, 86]. In the period from the initial stabilization of the condition and management of sepsis, carefully was initiated total parenteral nutrition (TPN) with gradual increase of the dose (up to 30 kcal/kg/daily, and protein 1.5-2.0 g/kg/daily) in order to be avoided electrolyte and metabolic disorders (the so called refeeding syndrome) [87, 88]. TPN ensures complete rest of GIT and minimizes the secretion from ECF. The enteral nutrition (EN) has some advantages before TPN, including maintenance of the enterohepatic circulation, intestinal function and structure, reduction of bacterial overgrowth, avoiding of complications related to the venous access.

Immediately when it becomes possible, careful administration of EN is initiated, with a small volume in the beginning, and gradual increase according to the tolerance, and without making the control over ECF unacceptable [82, 87, 88]. Feeding tube can be placed - distally from the fistule - upon proximally located ECF. In case of distally located ECF (distal ileum or colon), EN can be performed orally or via gastric tube. Another possibility for nutritional maintenance is the placement of nutritional tube under X-ray control directly in the fistula (fistuloclysis) [89, 90]. With the purpose of decrease of secretion and motility of GIT, as well as facilitation of the care for the wound in patients with ECF, sandostatin is administered (long-acting analogue of somatostatin), 100 µg subcutaneously three times daily. In patients in which no significant decrease of the production of ECF is observed after therapeutic course of 5-8 days, discontinuation of the administration of sandostatin is recommended [89, 90]. Another possibility for the wound care is the use of system for negative pressure (the so called vacuum assisted closure (VAC) system) [91, 92]. For performing of effective care for the wound, a multidisciplinary team of specialists is necessary [82].

Determination of the Morphological and Functional Characteristics of ECF

Determination of the morphological and functional characteristics of ECF is of exceptional significance for the proper choice of tactics for treatment. For this purpose, the medical history, the character of leaking intestinal content, and the condition of skin around the fistula (presence of maceration) are studied in details. The anatomical location of ECF, the condition of incoming and outgoing intestinal loop (presence of stenosis, obstruction), interrelation of the intestine, where the fistula is situated, and the adjacent organs, establishing the presence and distribution of purulent process (abscesses) in the abdominal cavity, are specified in details by means of endoscopic, echographic, computed tomographical (CT) and magnetic resonance imaging (MRI) examination, fistulography, examination of intestinal passage with contrast substance [76, 81, 83, 95, 96].

Plan for Definitive Therapy

Based on data from the literature in 5-20% of patients with ECF, spontaneous closure of the fistula is observed, while these are predominantly patients with low producing ECF without obstruction of passage distally, and concomitant septic complications. Upon absence of spontaneous closure of ECF during the first four weeks after their occurrence, it is proceeded to surgical treatment [75, 77, 81, 83, 96].

After making of a decision for performing of surgical intervention, a precise plan for intraoperative (positioning of patient on the operating table, preparation of the abdominal wall for minimization of direct contact with the intestinal content from ECF, a choice of operative access, primary intestinal anastomosis with/without cleaning enterostomy, etc.), and postoperative activities. It is also important to be determined the moment for performing of the surgical intervention [83, 95]. The early operative intervention (immediately after diagnosis making) is indicated only in patients with ECF and severe intraabdominal infection or intestinal obstruction. In this case, the conservative treatment is used for short-term preoperative preparation. In the rest patients surgical intervention is performed after a period of conservative treatment (about 6 weeks to 3 months) for stabilization of patient's condition, management of infection, correction of aqueous electrolyte disturbances, improvement of nutritional state [77, 81].

The population of patients with ECG is exceptionally heterogeneous. For optimal treatment of each patient individual plan is developed, which has as its purpose improvement of results and is of particular significance for the outcome of disease.

The treatment of patients with ECF is a clinical problem of current interest, because it remains a lot of contradictory and unsolved questions concerning the diagnostics, tactics, and methods of treatment, related to a continuous hospital stay and major economic costs.

Summarizing the literature data, it is to be noted that in the large intestinal fistulas most authors adhere to conservative treatment with thorough care for the wound and surrounding skin, while upon formation of small intestinal fistula, bypass anastomosis is recommended. When small intestinal and large intestinal fistulas are combined, the surgical tactics is determined by the location of the small intestinal fistula. In combined intestinal fistulas, including organs outside of GIT (e.g., urinary bladder, uterus) the surgical tactics must be determined by the morphological and functional characteristics of the intestinal fistula. At the time of closure of major defects of abdominal wall, the surgeon must be aware with the possibility for intraabdominal hypertension (the so call abdominal compartment syndrome) [97]. The average time from the appearing of ECF – part of the so-called "intestinal failure syndrome" to its definitive operative recovery is 6 months (in the range up to 28 months) [77]. The application of modern therapy with negative pressure with isolation of the fistula segment gives very good therapeutic results. The great diversity of ECF requires at the time of choosing of treatment to be applied individual approach for every particular patient. The recovery of integrity of GIT is a major factor for social and working rehabilitation of patients with ECF.

METHODS

Participants

Prospectively (in 7 cases, and retrospectively (in 27 cases), were analyzed (clinically and based on documents) 34 patients with established postoperative peritonitis at Department of Surgery, together with the Second Clinic of Anesthesia and Intensive Care of University Hospital Alexandrovska, Sofia (Bulgaria) for the last five years. Statistical methods from the pack SPSS for Windows 13.0 were used.

Results

Detailed history of the previous surgery was reported by patient and provided by the available documents. The basic pathology, general condition of patients, and degree of seriousness of peritonitis upon the first surgery, are determined as etiological risk factors. A connection between the emergency order at the first surgical intervention and the postoperative peritonitis was also proved.

The greater part of patients were in the average age group of 56.35 ± 6.01. The average age of patients, who had lethal outcome, was found to be 69.33 ± 5.14, while the average age of patients, who survived was 45.18 ± 3.72. The greater part of patients were men – 23 (67.6%), while women were 11 (32.4%).

The data for the etiology and characteristics of the initial surgical intervention in patients are given on the following Table 3.

The greater part of primary surgical interventions were related to procedures on colon and rectum – 18, while 67% of them were patients with malignant disease (50% malignant neoplasia in all 34 patients). Interesting as primary nosology are also one patient with extirpation of retroperitoneal tumour, one – with ovarian carcinoma, and one after peritoneal dialysis in terminal phase of chronic kidney disease. In three patients, the reason for the initial operation was severe necrotic pancreatitis, while in one – perforation of small intestine by a swallowed foreign body. In 12 patients – 35.3% the initial operation was in emergency order, while diffuse peritonitis was established in 6 of patients (17.6%), and total – in 3 (8.8%).

In etiological regard, the causes for development of postoperative peritonitis and the reasons for relaparotomy are as follows (Table 4):

In three patients the primary surgical intervention and the complication associated with it, which was a reason for relaparotomy, was performed in another health care institution. As a leading cause, dehiscence of surgical wound was outlined – 31.1%. Not every dehiscence however is accompanied by postoperative peritonitis. In this case patients with dehiscence of surgical wound were reflected – they had:

- preceding laceration of the sutured fascial layer, infection of the site of surgery, namely – suppuration of surgical wound;
- dehiscence with duration of more than 6 hours, in which secondary contamination of peritoneal cavity occurred and development of infectious inflammatory process over the visceral and parietal peritoneum.

Table 3. History of the primary surgical intervention

N	Localisation	Stomach/ duodenum	Pancreas/ gallbladder/ bile ducts	Jejunum/ ileum	Appendix	Colon/ rectum	Other	Total	Number of lethal outcomes
1	Primary pathology:	1	7	3	2	18	1(retroperitoneal tumor)+1(ovarian carcinoma)+1(peritoneal dialysis)	34	12
	-perforation		1	1	1	1		4	2
	-other	1	3	2	1	5	1	13	5
	-malignant neoplasm		3			12	2	17	5
2	Peritonitis:		1		2			12	5
	-local				2			3	
	-diffuse		2			3	1	6	3
	-total		1	1			1	3	2
3	Procedure:								
	- primary suture of perforation/lesion	1	1	1		1		4	
	- primary resection with anastomosis		1	2		12	1	16	
	-other (extirpation, necrectomy, ectomy of organ, stomia, etc.)		5		2	5	2	14	
4	Type of primary operation:								
	-elective	1	3	1	1	15	1	22	
	-emergency		4	2	1	3	2	12	

Table 4. Etiology of the cases of postoperative peritonitis

Cause	Number
Insufficiency of suture of large intestine	1
Insufficiency of suture of duodenum	1
Dehiscence of surgical wound	14
Persistent (tertiary postoperative) peritonitis after cholecystectomy and revision of extrahepatic bile ducts	1
Compartment syndrome and persistent (tertiary postoperative) peritonitis after necrotic pancreatitis (necrectomy and external biliary drainage)	3
Insufficiency of colo-rectal anastomosis	3
Insufficiency of colo-colonic anastomosis	3
Insufficiency of entero-enteral anastomosis	1
Insufficiency of anastomosis of extrahepatic bile ducts – bilio-biliary anastomosis	1
Insufficiency of anastomosis of extrahepatic bile ducts – bilio-digestive anastomosis	1
Insufficiency ("sinking") of colostoma after persistent (tertiary postoperative) peritonitis upon perforative diverticulitis	1
Secondary postoperative peritonitis after partial extirpation of locally advanced ovarian carcinoma with necroses and lysis	1
Mesenterial rethrombosis with necrosis and insufficiency of ileo-transversal anastomosis	1
Unspecified iatrogenic lesion/absence of serous membranes of intestine at the primary operation	4
Iatrogenic lesion of extrahepatic bile ducts	1
Abdominocentesis and fractionated peritoneal lavage due to chronic kidney disease	1
Postoperative interintestinal abscess	2
Postoperative ileo-psoas abscess	1
Postoperative retroperitoneal phlegmon (after necrotic pancreatitis)	1
Failure of clip of cystic duct after laparoscopic cholecystectomy	1 (relaparoscopy)
Postoperative perforation of stress-ulcus	1
Subhepatic abscess after relaparotomy near postoperative strangulation ileus	1
Totally	44 relaparotomies
	1 relaparoscopy

Table 5. Clinical cases with performed two relaparotomies in each patient

N	Patient - sex	Age	Diagnosis	Operation	Post-Operative Day	Lethal outcome before POD 30
9	female	63	Postoperative total peritonitis. Phlegmon of abdominal wall. State after laparotomies and colostomies du to total fibrinopurulent peritonitis and perforative pericolic abscess, and due to perforative diverticulitis.	Relaparotomy. Debridement, necrectomy, correction of colostomy, lavage, drainage Laparotomy - mesh, necrectomy, parastomal marsupialization.	3 3	-
21	male	69	Postoperative local peritonitis. Interintestinal hematoma and abscess. State after right-sided hemicolectomy. Right-sided ileo-psoas abscess.	Relaparotomy, evacuation of abscess lavage, drainage Rerelaparotomy, general debridement, evacuation of abscess, Resection of the wall of small intestine. Ileostomy, lavage, drainage	5 22	-
22	male	76	Postoperative local peritonitis. State after resection of sigmoid colon by the Hartmann's operation due to mesenteric thrombosis. Dehiscence of surgical wound. ═══════════ Dehiscence of surgical wound.	Relaparotomy, debridement. Lavage, drainage. Serclage. Re-relaparotomy. Lavage, drainage. Serclage.	4 7	+

Table 5. (Continued)

N	Patient - sex	Age	Diagnosis	Operation	Post-Operative Day	Lethal outcome before POD 30
31	female	59	Postoperative total peritonitis. State after pancreatic necrectomy and cholecystectomy, and transcystic drainage due to necrotic pancreatitis. Relapse of necrotic pancreatitis. Systemic inflammatory response syndrome (SIRS)-sepsis Persistent total postoperative peritonitis along with retroperitoneal phlegmon	Relaparotomy. Necrectomy, lavage, drainage. Re-relaparotomy. Revision of retroperitoneal space and evacuation of phlegmon. Lavage, drainage.	19 26	+

Table 6. Clinical cases with performed three re-laparotomies in every patient

N	Patient - sex	age	diagnosis	Operation	Post-Operative Day	Lethal outcome before POD 30
5	male	35	Total peritonitis. Compartment syndrome. State aster laparotomy due to necrotic pancreatitis, necrectomies and revision of gallbladder.	Relaparotomy, bursal and retroperitoneal revision, necrectomy, cleaning of small intestines, lavage, drainage. Secclage. Re-relaparotomy. lavage. Tracheostomy. Re-re-laparotomy. "Etappenlavage"	2 5 6	-
26	male	42	Diffuse postoperative peritonitis. State after hepatic common jejunal anastomosis. Insufficiency of anastomosis. Entero-cutaneal fistula and laparostomy. SIRS-sepsis. Entero-cutaneal fistula and laparostomy. SIRS-sepsis.	Relaparotomy. Revision of surgical wound. Suture of ileum. Lavage, drainage. Re-relaparotomy. Suture of small intestine. Resection of small intestine and ileo-ileal anastomosis. Kehr-drainage. Laparostomy. Revision of surgical wound. Suture of fistula. Lavage, correction and reposition of drainages.	58 41 15	+
30	female	67	Total postoperative peritonitis. State after rectal anterior resection and loop-ileostomy. Insufficiency of anastomosis.	Relaparotomy. Colostomy. Lavage, drainage. Serclage. Revision of surgical wound, necrectomy. Tracheostomy. Revision of surgical wound, necrectomy.	4 9 14	-

Table 6. (Continued)

N	Patient - sex	age	diagnosis	Operation	Post-Operative Day	Lethal outcome before POD 30
33	male	72	Diffuse peritonitis. State after right-sided hemicolectomy. Dehiscence of surgical wound. Persistent diffuse postoperative peritonitis. Perforative stress-ulcus of stomach. Dehiscence of surgical wound. Interintestinal abscess.	Relaparotomy, debridement, lavage, drainage. Serclage. Re-relaparotomy. Suture of ulcer. Ileo-transverse deanastomosis, ileostomy and transversostomy. Re-re-relaparotomy. Debridement, evacuation of interintestinal abscess. Lavage, drainage. Serclage.	11 1 5	+
34	female	40	Diffuse postoperative peritonitis. State after right-sided hemicolectomy. Laparotomy and relaparotomy due to strangulation ileus. Subhepatic abscess. Persistent total postoperative peritonitis. SIRS-sepsis. Dehiscence of surgical wound.	Re-relaparotomy. Debridement. Evacuation of subhepatic abscess. Ileostomy. Re-re-relaparotomy. Debridement. Resection of ileo-transverse anastomosis. Ileostomal correction.	17 6	+

The total number of operative reinterventions was 45-44 relaparotomies and 1 relaparoscopy due to "failure" of a clip after laparoscopic cholecystectomy; while during relaparoscopy, undertaken before the 24th hour from the primary operation, a new clip was placed - lavage and drainage was performed, with which the complication was managed by means of minimally invasive procedure. In four patients, re-relaparotomies were performed due to failure of management of the source of infection or newly occurred complication (Table 5):

Two of them had lethal outcome by Day 30 after the re-relaparotomy.

In 5 patients performing of third re-laparotomy (re-re-relaparotomy) became necessary due to impossible management of intraabdominal infection and additional complications (Table 6).

Three patients had lethal outcome by Day 30 after the last operative intervention.

In the tactics of operative treatment were used the described above principles for liquidation of septic focus, sanative treatment of peritoneal cavity, decompression and treatment/prevention of persistent or relapsing infection. In the most numerous dehiscences of surgical wound was applied serclage with the use of metalized, impregnated with silicone sutures - Ventrofil™. Postoperative fractionated transdrainage lavage of up to 48-72 hours was used in 3 patients, 2 of whom had lethal outcome. The preferred by us tactics is on demand relaparotomy. In two patients with total postoperative peritonitis – one based on necrotic pancreatitis, and one – with insufficiency of bilio-digestive anastomosis, tactics was used of planned relaparotomies, after placement of provisory sutures and prosthetic meshes. In two patients, the systemic extreme inflammatory response and the septic condition resulted in multisystem organ failure and lethal outcome. The technique of laparostomy, with daily sanative treatment of peritoneal cavity, was applied in three patients in severe condition, generalized peritonitis and SIRS-sepsis: a biliary peritonitis, in another case (based on necrotic pancreatitis) – both of them had lethal outcome - and a third case with feculent peritonitis at the large intestinal stomal insufficiency and dehiscence of surgical wound, in which healing was achieved.

Totally, for the whole group of postoperative peritonitis, the early postoperative mortality was registered in 13 patients – 38.2%.

DISCUSSION

The development of postoperative peritonitis continued to be not infrequently encountered and life-threatening complication (lethal outcome in 13 of the studied patients – 38.2%). The generalized forms – diffuse and total postoperative peritonitis are a serious cause for occurrence and worsening of SIRS-sepsis with multidrug resistant polymicrobial flora and multisystem organ failure. The diagnosis making of this complication is frequently hard even for an experienced surgical team. The qualitative and degree atypicality in the manifestation of clinical signs of peritonitis is a characteristic feature in its development in the early postoperative period. The strict interdisciplinary active dynamical observation and monitoring of patient is the key for the timely diagnosis making. The mortality is determined by four factors: inability to be controlled the radical septic source and to be liquidated the intraabdominal infection – septic abdomen (correlating with high Acute Physiology and Chronic Health Evacuation (APACHE) II score), advanced age, poor performance state, and condition of unconsciousness, groundless delay of relaparotomy. Only the more aggressive approach before the occurrence of sepsis could reduce the mortality and morbidity. Our opinion adheres to that of most authors: the decision for timely (in most cases "early") relaparotomy appears as a leading moment in the treatment of generalized postoperative peritonitis. The principles of surgical tactics – control of infection, sanative treatment of peritoneal cavity, decompression, averting of persistent infection – are to be pedantically observed; they are clearly defined and generally accepted, despite the nuances in the practical application of each of them in the different centres. There are a still some disputable questions, of which the searching of answers will continue in future time: Whether to be used on demand or planned relaparotomy; whether to be closed primarily the abdominal wall or to be proceeded to "etappenlavage" or laparostomy, especially through timely and adequate application of negative pressure therapy; how many and what type of drainages are to be used; where to be situated and how to be managed; when to be removed. The answer to all these questions must be achieved by obtaining high-level qualitative data from future prospective randomized controlled clinical trials.

REFERENCES

[1] Buchler MW, Baer HU, Brugger LE, Feodorovici MA Uhl W, Seiler C: [Surgical therapy of diffuse peritonitis: debridement and intraoperative extensive lavage]. *Chirurg* 1997;68:811-815.

[2] Pacelli F, Doglietto GB, Alfieri S, Piccioni E, Sgadari A, Gui D, Crucitti F: Prognosis in intra-abdominal infections. Multivariate analysis on 604 patients. *Arch Surg* 1996;131:641-645.

[3] Anderson ID, Fearon KC, Grant IS: Laparotomy for ab dominal sepsis in the critically ill. *Br J Surg* 1996;83:535-539.

[4] McLauchlan GJ, Anderson ID, Grant IS, Fearon KC: Outcome of patients with abdominal sepsis treated in an intensive care unit. *Br J Surg* 1995;82:524-529.

[5] Bader F. G., Schröder M., Kujath P., Muhl E, Bruch H. P., Eckmann C: Diffuse postoperative peritonitis – value of diagnostic parameters and impact of early indications for relaparotomy. *Eur J Med Res* (2009) 14: 491-496.

[6] van Ruler O, Lamme B, Gouma DJ, Reitsma JB, Boermeester MA: Variables associated with positive findings at relaparotomy in patients with secondary peritonitis. *Crit Care Med* 2007;35:468-476.

[7] Makela J, Kairaluoma MI: Relaparotomy for postoperative intra-abdominal sepsis in jaundiced patients. *Br J Surg* 1988;75:1157-1159.

[8] Mulier S, Penninckx F, Verwaest C, Filez L, Aerts R, Fieuws S, Lauwers P: Factors affecting mortality in generalized postoperative peritonitis: multivariate analysis in 96 patients. *World J Surg* 2003;27:379-384.

[9] Bosscha K, van Vroonhoven TJMV, van der Werken C. Surgical management of severe secondary peritonitis. Review. *Br. J. Surg.* 1999;86: 1371–1377.

[10] Parc Y, Frileux P, Schmitt G, et al. Management of postoperative peritonitis after anterior resection. Experience from a referral intensive care unit. *Dis. Colon Rectum* 2000;43:579–589.

[11] Hau T, Ohmann C, Wolmershäuser A, et al. Planned relaparotomy vs relaparotomy on demand in the treatment of intra-abdominal infections. *Arch. Surg.* 1995;130:1193–1197.

[12] Lévy E, Frileux P, Parc R, et al. Péritonites post-opératoires. Données communes. *Ann. Chir.* 1985;39:603–612.

[13] Wittmann DH, Aprahamian C, Bergstein JM. Etappenlavage. Advanced diffuse peritonitis managed by planned multiple laparotomies utilizing zippers, slide fastener, and Velcro analogue for temporary abdominal closure. *World J. Surg.* 1990;14:218–226.

[14] Bartels H, Barthlen W, Siewert JR. Therapie-ergebnisse der program mierten relaparotomie bei der diffusen peritonitis. *Chirurg* 1992;63: 174–180.

[15] Billing A, Fröhlich D, Mialkowskyj O, et al. Peritonitisbehandlung mit der etappenlavage (EL): prognosekriterien und behandlungsverlauf. *Langenbecks Arch. Chir.* 1992;377:305–313. [*Peritonitis treatment with stage lavage (EL): prognostic criteria and course of treatment.*]

[16] Pusajó JF, Bumaschny E, Doglio GR, et al. Postoperative intraabdominal sepsis requiring reoperation. Value of a predictive index. *Arch. Surg.* 1993;128:218–223.

[17] Lévy E, Cugnenc PH, Parc R, et al. Péritonites post-opératoires par lésion de l'intestin grêle. A propos de 217 cas. *Ann. Chir.* 1985;39:631–641. [Postoperative peritonitis due to lesion of the small intestine. About 217 cases.]

[18] Kerremans R, Penninckx F, Lauwers P, et al. Mortality of generalised peritonitis patients reduced by planned relaparotomies. Intensivmed. Notfallmed. A*nästhesiol*. 1982;37:104–107.

[19] Penninckx FM, Kerremans RP, Lauwers PM. Planned relaparotomies in the surgical treatment of severe generalised peritonitis from intestinal origin. *World J. Surg.* 1983;7:762–766.

[20] Penninckx F, Kerremans R, Filez L, et al. Planned relaparotomies for advanced, established peritonitis from colonic origin. *Acta Chir. Belg.* 1990;90:269–274.

[21] Kern E, Klaue P, Arbogast R. Programmierte peritoneal-lavage bei diffuser peritonitis. *Chirurg* 1983;54:306–310.

[22] Hay JM, Duchatelle P, Elman A, et al. The abdomen left open. *Chirurgie* 1979;105:508–510.

[23] Sakai L, Daake J, Kaminski DL. Acute perforation of sigmoid diverticuli. *Am. J. Surg.* 1981;142:12–16.

[24] Andrus C, Doering M, Herrmann VM, et al. Planned reoperation for generalized intraabdominal infection. *Am. J. Surg.* 1986;152:682–686.

[25] Van Goor H, Hulsebos RG, Blechrodt RP. Complications of planned relaparotomy in patients with severe general peritonitis. *Eur. J. Surg.* 1997;163:61–66.

[26] Sautner T, Gotzinger P, Redl Wenzl EM, et al. Does reoperation for abdominal sepsis enhance the inflammatory host response? *Arch. Surg.* 1997;132:250–255.

[27] Schein M. Planned reoperations and open management in critical intraabdominal infections: prospective experience in 52 cases. *World J. Surg.* 1991;15:537–545.

[28] Schein M, Saadia R, Decker GGA. The open management of the septic abdomen. *Surg. Gynecol. Obstet.* 1986;163:587–592.

[29] Wacha H, Linder MM, Feldman U, WeschG, Gundlach E, Steifensand RA. Mannheim peritonitis index - prediction of risk of death from peritonitis: construction of a statistical and validation of an empirically based index. *Theoretical Surg* 1987; 1: 169-77.

[30] Dupont H: The empiric treatment of nosocomial intra-abdominal infections. *Int J Infect Dis* 2007, 11(S1):S1-S6. PubMed Abstract | Publisher Full Text.

[31] Harbarth S, Uckay I: Are there any patients with peritonitis who require empiric therapy for enterococcus? *Eur J Microbiol Infect Dis* 2004, 23:73-77. Publisher Full Text.

[32] Chromik AM, Meiser A, Hölling J, et al.: Identification of patients at risk for development of tertiary peritonitis on a surgical intensive care unit. *J Gastrointest Surg* 2009, 13:1358-1367. PubMed Abstract | Publisher Full Text.

[33] Herzog T., Uhl W. (2018) Postoperative Peritonitis: Etiology, Diagnosis, and Treatment. In: Sartelli M., Bassetti M., Martin-Loeches I. (eds) *Abdominal Sepsis. Hot Topics in Acute Care Surgery and Trauma.* Springer, Cham. https://doi.org/10.1007/978-3-319-59704-1_12.

[34] Shah A: Postoperative Peritonitis. *The I-net J Surg,* Vol. 6 N.2, http://ispub.com/IJS/6/2/10390#.

[35] Pollock AV. Non operative anti-infective treatment of Intra abdominal infection. *World J Surg* 1990; 14:227-230.

[36] Farthmann EH, Schoffel U. Principles and limitations of operative management of intra-abdominal infection. *World J Surg* 1990; 14:210-17.

[37] Lennard ES, Dellinger EP, Wertz MJ. Implications of leukocytosis and fever at conclusion of antibiotic therapy for intraabdominal sepsis. *Ann Surg 1982*; 19:195.

[38] Lagarde MC, Bolton Js, Conn I. Intraperitoneal povidone iodine in experimental peritonitis. *Ann Surg* 1978; 187:613.

[39] Hallerback, Andersson C, et al. Prospective randomized study of continous peritoneal lavage post operatively in the treatment of purulent peritonitis. *Surg Gynec Obstetr* 1986; 163: 433-36.

[40] Duff JH, Moffar J. Abdominal sepsis managed by leaving abdomen open. *Surg* 1981; 90:774-78.

[41] Anderson AD, Mandelbaum DM. Open packing of peritoneal cavity in generalized bacterial peritonitis. *Amer J Surg* 1983; 145:131-35.

[42] Raith EP, Udy AA, Bailey M, McGloughlin S, MacIsaac C, Bellomo R, Pilcher DV, for the Australian and New Zealand Intensive Care Society (ANZICS) Centre for Outcomes and Resource Evaluation

(CORE) (2017) Prognostic accuracy of the SOFA score, SIRS criteria, and qSOFA score for in-hospital mortality among adults with suspected infection admitted to the intensive care unit. *JAMA* 317:290. https://doi.org/10.1001/jama.2016. 20328.

[43] Das K, Ozdogan M, Karateke F, Uzun AS, Sozen S, Ozdas S (2014) Comparison of APACHE II, P-POSSUM and SAPS II scoring systems in patients underwent planned laparotomies due to secondary peritonitis. *Ann Ital Chir* 85:16–21. PMID: 24755836.

[44] Vincent JL, Moreno R, Takala J et al. (1996) The SOFA (Sepsis-related Organ Failure Assessment) score to describe organ dysfunction/failure. *Intensive Care Med* 22:707–710. https://doi.org/10. 1007/BF01709751.

[45] Kologlu M, Elker D, Altun H, Sayek I (2001) Validation of MPI and PIA II in two different groups of patients with secondary peritonitis. *Hepatogastroenterology*.;48:147–51. PMID: 11268952.

[46] Biondo S, Ramos E, Fraccalvieri D, Kreisler E, Ragué JM, Jaurrieta E (2006) Comparative study of left colonic Peritonitis Severity Score and Mannheim Peritonitis Index. *Br J Surg* 93:616–622. https://doi.org/10.1002/bjs.5326.

[47] Møller MH, Engebjerg MC, Adamsen S, Bendix J, Thomsen RW (2012) The Peptic Ulcer Perforation (PULP) score: a predictor of mortality following peptic ulcer perforation. A cohort study. *Acta Anaesthesiol Scand* 56:655–662. https://doi.org/10.1111/j.1399-6576.2011.02609.x.

[48] Sartelli M, Abu-Zidan FM, Catena F, Griffiths EA, Di Saverio S, Coimbra R, et al. (2015) Global validation of the WSES Sepsis Severity Score for patients with complicated intraabdominal infections: a prospective multicenter study (WISS Study). *World J Emerg Surg* 10:61 https://doi.org/10.1186/s13017-015-0055-0.

[49] Rhodes A, Phillips G, Beale R, Cecconi M, Chiche JD, et al. The Surviving Sepsis Campaign bundles and outcome: results from the International Multicentre Prevalence Study on Sepsis (the IMPreSS study). *Intensive Care Med.* 2015 Sep;41(9):1620-8. doi: 10.1007/s00134-015-3906-y. Epub 2015 Jun 25. PMID: 26109396.

[50] Seymour CW, Gesten F, Prescott HC, Friedrich ME, Iwashyna TJ, et al. Time to Treatment and Mortality during Mandated Emergency Care for Sepsis. *N Engl J Med*. 2017 Jun 8;376(23):2235-2244. doi: 10.1056/NEJMoa1703058. Epub 2017 May 21. PMID: 28528569; PMCID: PMC5538258.

[51] Sartelli M, Chichom-Mefire A, Labricciosa FM, Hardcastle T, Abu-Zidan FM, et al. The management of intra-abdominal infections from a global perspective: 2017 WSES guidelines for management of intra-abdominal infections. *World J Emerg Surg*. 2017 Jul 10;12:29. doi: 10.1186/s13017-017-0141-6. Erratum in: *World J Emerg Surg*. 2017 Aug 2;12 :36. PMID: 28702076; PMCID: PMC5504840.

[52] Solomkin JS, Mazuski JE, Bradley JS, Rodvold KA, Goldstein EJ, et al. Diagnosis and management of complicated intra-abdominal infection in adults and children: guidelines by the Surgical Infection Society and the Infectious Diseases Society of America. *Clin Infect Dis*. 2010 Jan 15;50(2):133-64. doi: 10.1086/649554. Erratum in: *Clin Infect Dis*. 2010 Jun 15;50(12):1695. Dosage error in article text. PMID: 20034345.

[53] Mazuski JE, Tessier JM, May AK, Sawyer RG, Nadler EP, et al. The Surgical Infection Society Revised Guidelines on the Management of Intra-Abdominal Infection. *Surg Infect* (Larchmt). 2017 Jan;18(1):1-76. doi: 10.1089/sur.2016.261. PMID: 28085573.

[54] Rhodes A, Evans LE, Alhazzani W, Levy MM, Antonelli M, et al. Surviving Sepsis Campaign: International Guidelines for Management of Sepsis and Septic Shock: 2016. *Intensive Care Med*. 2017 Mar;43(3):304-377. doi: 10.1007/s00134-017-4683-6. Epub 2017 Jan 18. PMID: 28101605.

[55] Tellor B, Skrupky LP, Symons W, High E, Micek ST, Mazuski JE. Inadequate source control and inappropriate antibiotics are key determinants of mortality in patients with intra-abdominal sepsis and associated bacteremia. *Surg Infect* (Larchmt). 2015;16:785–93. doi: 10.1089/sur.2014.166. Epub 2015 Aug 10. PMID: 26258265.

[56] Bryan P White, Jamie L Wagner, Katie E Barber, Travis King, Kayla R Stover. Risk factors for failure in complicated intraabdominal

infections. *SMJ* 2018;111:125-132. doi:10.14423/SMJ.000000000 0000770.

[57] De Waele JJ. Early source control in sepsis. *Langenbecks Arch Surg.* 2010 Jun;395(5):489-94. doi: 10.1007/s00423-010-0650-1. Epub 2010 Jun 2. *PMID:* 20517699.

[58] Leppäniemi A, Kimball EJ, De Laet I et al. (2015) Management of abdominal sepsis—a paradigm shift? *Anestezjol Intense Ter* 47:400–408. doi:10.5603/AIT.a2015.0026.

[59] Opal, Steven M. MD Source Control in Sepsis Urgent or Not So Fast? *Critical Care Medicine*: 2017, 45(1):130-132. doi: 10.1097/ccm.0000000000002123

[60] Coccolini F, Montori G, Ceresoli M, Catena F, Ivatury R, et al. IROA: International Register of Open Abdomen, preliminary results. *World J Emerg Surg.* 2017 Feb 21;12:10. doi: 10.1186/s13017-017-0123-8. Erratum in: *World J Emerg Surg.* 2017 Mar 9;12 :13. PMID: 28239409; PMCID: PMC5320725.

[61] Quyn AJ, Johnston C, Hall D, Chambers A, Arapova N, Ogston S, Amin AI. (2012) The open abdomen and temporary abdominal closure systems - historical evolution and systematic review. *Colorectal Dis* 14:e429–e438.

[62] Demetriades D, Salim A. Management of the open abdomen. *Surg Clin North Am.* 2014 Feb;94(1):131-53. doi: 10.1016/j.suc.2013.10.010. PMID: 24267502.

[63] Regner JL, Kobayashi L, Coimbra R. Surgical strategies for management of the open abdomen. *World J Surg.* 2012 Mar;36(3):497-510. doi: 10.1007/s00268-011-1203-7. PMID: 21847684.

[64] Marshall JC. Intra-abdominal infections. *Microbes Infect.* 2004 Sep;6(11):1015-25. doi: 10.1016/j.micinf.2004.05.017. PMID: 15345234.

[65] Sartelli M, Weber DG, Ruppé E, Bassetti M, Wright BJ, et al. Antimicrobials: a global alliance for optimizing their rational use in intra-abdominal infections (AGORA). *World J Emerg Surg.* 2016 Jul 15;11:33. doi: 10.1186/s13017-016-0089-y. Erratum in: *World J*

Emerg Surg. 2017 Aug 2;12 :35. PMID: 27429642; PMCID: PMC4946132.

[66] Sartelli M, Catena F, Abu-Zidan FM, Ansaloni L, Biffl WL, et al. Management of intra-abdominal infections: recommendations by the WSES 2016 consensus conference. *World J Emerg Surg.* 2017 May 4;12:22. doi: 10.1186/s13017-017-0132-7. PMID: 28484510; PMCID: PMC5418731.

[67] De Waele JJ. Abdominal Sepsis. Curr Infect Dis Rep. 2016 Aug;18(8):23. doi: 10.1007/s11908-016-0531-z. PMID: 27363829.

[68] Vincent JL. Give your patient a fast hug (at least) once a day. *Crit Care Med.* 2005 Jun;33(6):1225-9. doi: 10.1097/01.ccm.000 0165962.16682.46. PMID: 15942334.

[69] Malbrain ML, Cheatham ML (2011) Definitions and pathophysiological implications of intra-abdominal hypertension and abdominal compartment syndrome. *Am Surg.* 77(Suppl 1):6–11.

[70] Kirkpatrick A, Roberts D, Waele J et al. (2013) Intra-abdominal hypertension and the abdominal compartment syndrome: updated consensus definitions and clinical practice guidelines from the World Society of the Abdominal Compartment Syndrome. *Intensive Care Med.* 39:1190-1206.

[71] Cheatham ML. (2009) Nonoperative management of intraabdominal hypertension and abdominal compartment syndrome. *World J Surg.* 33:1116–1122.

[72] De Keulenaer BL, De Waele JJ, Malbrain ML (2011) Nonoperative management of intra-abdominal hypertension and abdominal compartment syndrome: evolving concepts. *Am Surg.* 77(Suppl 1):S34–S41.

[73] De Waele J, Desender L, De Laet I, Ceelen W, Pattyn P, Hoste E. (2010) Abdominal decompression for abdominal compartment syndrome in critically ill patients: a retrospective study. *Acta Clin Belg.* 65:399–403.

[74] De Waele JJ, Hoste EA, Malbrain ML. (2006) Decompressive laparotomy for abdominal compartment syndrome—a critical analysis. *Crit Care.* 10(2):R51.

[75] Lundy JB, Fischer JE. Historical perspectives in the care of patients with enterocutaneous fistula. *Clin Colon Rectal Surg.* 2010;23(3):133-141.

[76] Mawdsley JE, Hollington P, Bassett P, Windsor AJ, Forbes A, Gabe SM. An analysis of predictive factors for healing and mortality in patients with enterocutaneous fistulas. *Aliment Pharmacol Ther* 2008;28(9):1111–1121.

[77] Hollington P, Mawdsley J, Lim W, Gabe SM, Forbes A, Windsor AJ. An 11-year experience of enterocutaneous fistula. *Br J Surg.* 2004;91(12):1646-1651.

[78] Lynch AC, Delaney CP, Senagore AJ, Connor JT, Remzi FH, Fazio VW. Clinical outcome and factors predictive of recurrence after enterocutaneous fistula surgery. *Ann Surg.* 2004;240(5):825-831.

[79] Jamie Murphy, Alexander Hotouras, Lena Koers, Chetan Bhan, Michael Glynn, Christopher L. Chan, Establishing a regional enterocutaneous fistula service: The Royal London hospital experience, *International Journal of Surgery*, Volume 11, Issue 9, 2013, Pages 952-956.

[80] McNaughton V, Brown J, Hoeflok J, et al. Summary of best practice recommendations for management of enterocutaneous fistulae from the Canadian Association for Enterostomal Therapy ECF Best Practice Recommendations Panel. *J Wound Ostomy Continence Nurs* 2010;37(2):173-184.

[81] Martinez JL, Luque-de-León E, Ballinas-Oseguera G, Mendez JD, Juárez-Oropeza MA, Román-Ramos R. Factors predictive of recurrence and mortality after surgical repair of enterocutaneous fistula. *Journal of Gastrointestinal Surgery.* 2012;16(1):156–164.

[82] Datta V, Engledow A, Chan S, Forbes A, Cohen CR, Windsor A. The management of enterocutaneous fistula in a regional unit in the United Kingdom: a prospective study. *Dis Colon Rectum.* 2010;53(2):192-199.

[83] Schecter WP, Hirshberg A, Chang DS, et al. Enteric fistulas: principles of management. *J Am Coll Surg.* 2009;209(4):484–491.

[84] Visschers RG, Olde Damink SW, Winkens B, Soeters PB, van Gemert WG. Treatment strategies in 135 consecutive patients with enterocutaneous fistulas. *World J Surg.* 2008;32(3):445-453.
[85] Dellinger RP, Levy MM, Rhodes A, et al. Surviving sepsis campaign: international guidelines for management of severe sepsis and septic shock: 2012. *Critical Care Medicine.* 2013;41:580–637.
[86] Solomkin JS, Mazuski JE, Bradley JS, et al. Diagnosis and management of complicated intra-abdominal infection in adults and children: guidelines by the Surgical Infection Society and the Infectious Diseases Society of America. *Clin Infect Dis* 2010;50(2):133–164.
[87] Bleier JIS, Hedrick T. Metabolic support of the enterocutaneous fistula patient. *Clinics in Colon and Rectal Surgery.* 2010;23(3):142–148.
[88] Kumpf VJ, de Aguilar-Nascimento JE, Diaz-Pizarro Graf JI, Hall AM, McKeever L, Steiger E, Winkler MF, Compher CW; FELANPE; American Society for Parenteral and Enteral Nutrition. ASPEN-FELANPE Clinical Guidelines& Nutrition Support of Adult patients with enterocutaneous Fistula. *JPEN J Parenter Enteral Nutr.* 2017 Jan;41(1):104-112. doi: 10.1177/0148607116680792.
[89] Lloyd DA, Gabe SM, Windsor AC. Nutrition and management of enterocutaneous fistula. *Br J Surg* 2006; 93(9):1045–1055.
[90] YinWu, Jianan Ren, Gefei Wang, Bo Zhou, Chao Ding, Guosheng Gu, Jun Chen, Song Liu, and Jieshou Li. Clinical Study Fistuloclysis Improves Liver Function and Nutritional Status in Patients with High-Output Upper Enteric Fistula. *Gastroenterology Research and Practice* Volume 2014, Article ID 941514, 10 pages http://dx.doi.org/10.1155/2014/941514.
[91] Teubner A, Morrison K, Ravishankar HR. Anderson ID, Scott NA, Carlson GL.. Fistuloclysis can successfully replace parenteral feeding in the nutritional support of patients with enterocutaneous fistula. *Br J Surg* 2004;91(5):625-631.
[92] Alivizatos V, Felekis D, Zorbalas A. Evaluation of the effectiveness of octreotide in the conservative treatment of postoperative

enterocutaneous fistulas. *Hepatogastroenterology* 2002;49(46):1010–1012.

[93] Hesse U, Ysebaert D, de Hemptinne B. Role of somatostatin- 14 and its analogues in the management of gastrointestinal fistulae: clinical data. *Gut* 2001;49(Suppl 4):iv11–iv21.

[94] Gunn LA, Follmar KE, Wong MS, Lettieri SC, Levin LS, Erdmann D. Management of enterocutaneous fistulas using negative-pressure dressings. *Ann Plast Surg* 2006;57(6): 621–625.

[95] Heller L, Levin SL, Butler CE. Management of abdominal wound dehiscence using vacuum assisted closure in patients with compromised healing. *Am J Surg* 2006;191(2):165–172.

[96] Martinez JL, Luque-de-Leon E, Mier J, Blanco-Benavides R, Robledo F. Systematic management of postoperative enterocutaneous fistulas: factors related to outcomes. *World J Surg.* 2008;32(3):436-444.

[97] Evenson AR, Fischer JE. Current management of enterocutaneous fistula. *J Gastrointest Surg.* 2006;10(3):455-464.

[98] Fischer JE. The importance of reconstruction of the abdominal wall after gastrointestinal fistula closure. *Am J Surg.* 2009;197(1):131-132.

In: Peritonitis
Editor: David F. Walker

ISBN: 978-1-53619-624-5
© 2021 Nova Science Publishers, Inc.

Chapter 2

PERITONITIS IN ASSISTED PERITONEAL DIALYSIS. RESULTS OF A CONSOLIDATED PROGRAM

Consolación Rosado-Rubio[1,*], *PhD, MD,*
Isabelle Brayer[2], *Carla Bernaer*[2], *Nadine Rossez*[2],
Elena Vieru[2], *Christelle Fosso*[2], *MD*
and Max Dratwa[2], *PhD, MD*

[1]Service of Nephrology. Ávila Hospital, SACYL, Ávila, Spain
[2]Peritoneal Dialysis Unit of the CHU Brugmann, Brussels, Belgium

ABSTRACT

Peritoneal dialysis is a main part of the treatment of the end-stage kidney disease. It offers results comparable to hemodialysis. It provides a home dialysis treatment, which offers some advantages in order to improve the patient's quality of life, mainly in elderly people. One of the most serious complications is peritonitis, which can lead to the technique failure and the patient's transfer to hemodialysis. Assisted peritoneal

---

[*] Ccorresponding Author's E-mail - crosadorubio@gmail.com.

dialysis is a peritoneal dialysis modality in which a nurse goes to the patient's home to perform the dialysis technique when the patient is unable to do it himself (elderly or disabled people) and there is a lack of family support.

We have studied the assisted peritoneal dialysis program of the CHU Brugmann, in Brussels, a consolidated program who was implemented many years ago, in order to know its organization, the way of performing the technique and the rate of peritonitis in this kind of peritoneal dialysis since the implantation of the technique in the hospital.

Assisted peritoneal dialysis in CHU Brugmann is supported by home-care companies, who provide the visiting nurses. The hospital has imposed a very strict training protocol to the visiting nurses, so the rate of peritonitis is weak (not superior to autonomous patients or patients helped by their family).

Assisted peritoneal dialysis in hospitals who have a consolidated program is a safe and valid way of performing an in-home treatment of the end-stage chronic kidney to avoid the transfer to hemodialysis in a sanitary facility.

BACKGROUND

Peritoneal dialysis is an integral part of the treatment scheme for end-stage kidney disease and its results are globally comparable to those of other dialysis modalities [1]. Its development began in the 70's, but in the 80's it broke into the usual clinical practice. These first experiences were marked by the high rate of infections in the peritoneal cavity (named peritonitis), which marked a very short survival of the technique. This was the cause of the little use of this technique for nearly 20 years [1, 2].

The incidence of peritonitis has evolved from several episodes per patient per year to about one episode per patient every two or more years [3]. This large decrease in the peritonitis rate is due to advances in the connection system, especially the use of the double bag system, prevention of infection of the catheter exit site and its daily care and a better training of patients and their caregivers [4-9]. New peritoneal dialysis solutions, which, being more biocompatible, improve the condition of peritoneal defense system, have also contributed to the decrease in the peritonitis rate [10]. Even so, it remains one of the main causes of the failure of the technique and of the patient's transfer (temporary or definitively) to hemodialysis [1, 2].

Staphylococci are the main causes of peritonitis associated with peritoneal dialysis, especially *S. epidermidis*, which causes the infection by contact contamination. *S. aureus* is frequently associated with infections of the catheter exit site and the subcutaneous tunnel [11]. Nowadays, we can see an increase in gram-negative bacilli infections [11, 12], which may be related to intestinal impairment and these germs penetrate the peritoneal cavity using a transmural route. Of them, *E. coli* is the most frequently involved agent, but its response to the treatment is good, unlike pseudomonas, which often require the catheter removal [11, 13]. Fungal peritonitis is rare [14], but it has a high morbidity and mortality. It is related to repeated antibiotic cycles and the most common species is *C. albicans*. Mycobacterias also cause peritonitis, but these are much rarer and their diagnosis is difficult because their growth in culture is very slow [15].

Peritonitis due to peritoneal dialysis can be suspected when the patient suffers from abdominal pain and has cloudy peritoneal fluid (due to the presence of leukocytes and, sometimes fibrin), which is the main and most early sign [7]. Abdominal pain may be absent, or it may have low intensity. Severe pain should make us think about an infection caused by gram-negative bacilli [12]. In the elderly, digestive symptoms are frequent [6]. In patients treated with automated peritoneal dialysis, turbidity of the drained fluid may be difficult to detect, due to the more frequent renewal of dialysis fluid in this technique [4].

For the diagnosis of peritonitis due to peritoneal dialysis, we need to determine the presence of leukocytes in the dialysate. We can use a reactive urine strip for doing that, but we must confirm the result with a cytological examination of the fluid (leukocytes > 100/mL with more than 50% of polynuclear cells after a permanence period of 2 hours) [5].

The confirmatory diagnosis is given by the cytological examination of the dialysate, that is to say, direct examination with Gram stain and dialysate culture in blood culture tubes. A negative culture does not exclude the diagnosis of a peritoneal infection.

The usefulness of abdominal X-ray focusing on the diaphragmatic domes in case of severe pain has been demonstrated for the diagnosis of a possible pneumoperitoneum, which may indicate the presence of a hollow viscera perforation [5-7].

In polymicrobial infections, abdominal tests such as colonoscopy, ultrasound, or CAT scan are advisable to look for an abdominal cause of these infections [12, 13].

It is not necessary to wait for the outcome of complementary tests to begin empirical antibiotic treatment.

There are certain cases in which infections are particularly difficult to eradicate, such as refractory, relapsing and recurrent peritonitis [11]. Refractory peritonitis is the persistence of a cloudy liquid after 5 days of appropriate antibiotic therapy. Except in some cases, it should lead to a rapid catheter ablation. The most common causative microorganisms are gram-negative bacilli, *S. aureus*, pseudomonas and fungi. Relapsing peritonitis occurs within four weeks of completing antibiotic treatment by a previous peritonitis and it is caused by the same germ. It usually indicates the presence of a biofilm in the catheter, so it is usually necessary to remove the catheter, although sometimes fibrinolysis is performed to try to remove the biofilm in an attempt to conserve the catheter [11]. Recurrent peritonitis is an infection that occurs within 4 weeks of having completed the antibiotic treatment of a previous episode, but it is produced by a different organism.

These particular cases are sometimes the cause of a temporary transfer to hemodialysis, but should not be considered a priori as indications of definitive transfer [11, 13]. A regular evaluation of the incidence of peritoneal infections in the hospital and a comparison with the standards ensures the quality of any peritoneal dialysis program [3, 8].

The use of mupirocin in the exit site of the catheter is useful to reduce the incidence of peritoneal infections by *S. aureus*. The application of gentamicin decreases the incidence of *S. aureus* and gram-negative bacilli infections [13].

When a peritonitis is suspected, empirical antibiotic therapy should be established early, even before obtaining the results of the peritoneal fluid examination [3]. Although the intraperitoneal route is the preferred mode of administration of antibiotics, there is no consensus on the rate of administration of them: fractionated in each bag or a single dose in a bag, although the latter option is the most frequently used [4, 5, 8].

The initial antibiotic therapy is empirical and it should be effective for staphylococci, gram-negative bacilli and pseudomonas. It should last at least 2 weeks, although sometimes it should be extended to 3 weeks to complete the treatment [11-13]. A combination of 1st generation cephalosporins or vancomycin is often used for gram-positive bacteria, with ceftazidime or amikacin for gram-negative bacteria. Cefazolin has been replaced by vancomycin in many hospitals, because of the high incidence of methicillin-resistant staphylococci or enterococci [11]. However, no specific pattern has been clearly shown to be superior to others and all of them need to be adapted to local ecology.

In addition to antibiotics, heparin should be systematically administered in the peritoneum, in order to prevent the formation of fibrin deposits and because heparin has some local anti-inflammatory effect [5]. In case of significant pain, it may be useful to carry out 2 to 3 successive exchanges with a short duration of stay, as a peritoneal wash. In some cases, peritoneal dialysis catheter removal and transitory (sometimes definitive) passage to hemodialysis are necessary, as in pseudomonas or fungal infections or in relapsing or refractory peritonitis [11].

Peritoneal dialysis is performed at the patient's home, by himself or his family or, in certain countries, by nurses who go to the patient's home several times per day, a modality called assisted peritoneal dialysis [9]. For the prevention of peritonitis, the education of the patient and the health care professionals or family members who will carry out the technique is essential [9, 16]. The length and frequency of the educational sessions vary widely in the different hospitals. However, a minimum of three sessions is likely to be required; in them, special attention should be paid to learning about the connection and disconnection system, since connections and disconnections are the most dangerous moments of the technique, in which infections are more probable [6, 8, 16].

Assisted peritoneal dialysis is performed in the patient's home by visiting nursing staff. This modality of peritoneal dialysis is spreading, mainly in some European countries, so it is necessary to establish a financing system [17], which differs according to the different sanitary systems, and a very strict training protocol in order to avoid complications of the technique, mainly peritonitis [16].

The first assisted peritoneal dialysis experiences took place in France in 1977, thanks to the commitment of the nursing home group and the implementation of a very attractive salary system. In Belgium, assisted peritoneal dialysis was implanted in 1996 [18]. This first experience lasted only 7 months, because of the death of the patient due to peritonitis secondary to a *colibacilus* [18].

In 1999, the first treatment of a patient was carried out by an organized group of home nurses in Belgium. In 2016, the new collaboration agreement between hospitals and home care services was established, with new modalities for the reimbursement of peritoneal dialysis treatments in Belgium [19], in order to encourage the assisted peritoneal dialysis over the hospital hemodialysis.

OBJECTIVES

We have studied the assisted peritoneal dialysis program of the CHU Brugmann (in Brussels, Belgium). We have performed a cross-sectional study of the patients included in this program in June 2018, which describes the type of patients and the results of the program, together with the study of the rate of peritonitis since the beginning of the assisted peritoneal dialysis. We want to know if these group of patients have the same demographic and social profile that other groups of patients who are included in this kind of treatment, and to assess if this modality of treatment is safe for the patient, focusing in the peritonitis rate.

PATIENTS AND METHODS

We have conducted an observational, descriptive and cross-sectional study of the demographic and clinical characteristics and the results of the assisted peritoneal dialysis of the group of patients included in the assisted peritoneal dialysis program in June 2018.

We have also studied the rate of peritonitis in assisted peritoneal dialysis from the beginning of the program in the hospital, comparing it with the autonomous and helped-by-relatives' modalities.

The data analysis was performed with the SPSS v.20.0 program for MacOS, the quantitative results are expressed as median (first and third quartile) and qualitative as a percentage.

We have collected data from the registries of the hospital, the patients' medical records and we have had many interviews with the nurses and the rest of the staff of the Peritoneal Dialysis Unit of the hospital, in order to know the organization of the program.

RESULTS

CHU Brugmann is located in the north of the city of Brussels (Belgium), an area with a large percentage of immigrant population. In 2018 it has 853 beds and a Nephrology-Dialysis Clinic with 37 haemodialysis places and 22 patients receiving peritoneal dialysis.

The Peritoneal Dialysis Unit is staffed by 3 full-time and one part-time nurses, who evaluate the patient's autonomy and decide which one of the peritoneal dialysis modalities offered in the hospital is best suited to them: autonomous, helped by the family or assisted peritoneal dialysis. They promote the autonomous mode, since it is less expensive and it allows the patient to take responsibility for their disease without overburdening their environment. If it is not feasible, family help is advocated, leaving the assisted peritoneal dialysis as the last option (because it is more expensive). The nurses who go to the patients' houses for performing the peritoneal dialysis to the patients belonging to this hospital work for home care agencies, they are not liberal nurses, since the strict protocol for avoiding peritonitis has stablished a ratio of 3 nurses per each patient, in order to assure the continuity of the nurse care in the case of holidays or casualties.

Nurses' tasks are: assembly, connection and disconnection of the cycler, manual exchanges, care of the catheter and the exit site, assistance in the collection of 24-hour urine for the medical consultation, management of the deposit of dialysis material with Baxter® and Fresenius® and resolution of the cycler alarm problems by telephone. They go to the patient's home several times a day, depending on the patient's degree of autonomy: if the patient performs the connection and disconnection of the cycler, the nurse goes once a day to weigh the patient, perform the care of the catheter and its exit site and assemble and disassemble the machine. If the patient is not autonomous and has no help from the environment (family members), the nurse visits him every morning and evening. Nurses must have a registry of all the patient's data and all the problems of the technique.

On the first visit to the patient's home, a nurse from the Peritoneal Dialysis Unit of the hospital accompanies them to supervise the work and check compliance with the protocol. Every 6 months there is a meeting at the headquarters of the companies with the nurses of the Peritoneal Dialysis Unit to discuss the clinical status of each patient and solve any problems that may arise.

The home-based staff who are going to take care of CHU Brugmann patients must, absolutely, be trained in the hospital, even if they already have knowledge of peritoneal dialysis. This requirement derives from the fact that these companies work with different hospitals, which have different protocols and this hospital requires strict monitoring of the patients. Thus, this staff performs an apprenticeship of 4 hours in 2 days in the Peritoneal Dialysis Unit: the first day, they receive theoretical training and the second day they receive practice training. The trained staff cannot teach the new one. Each year there are one or two days of continuing training between the nurses of the hospital and the nurses of the home care services companies, in order to remind them the key concepts. Even so, the patient and his family are trained in the connection and disconnection of the cycler, in order to manage immediate emergencies.

Since the beginning of the assisted peritoneal dialysis in Belgium, 86 patients have performed this modality of peritoneal dialysis in CHU Brugmann. They had a median age of 66.5 years (60-76.75). A slight predominance of males was observed: 48 men (55.8%) compared to 38 women (44.2%). In figure 1 we can see the graphical representation of the distribution of the different modalities of peritoneal dialysis in this hospital since the beginning of it. The autonomous modality is the most used, followed by the help of the family members and, in the last place, assisted peritoneal dialysis.

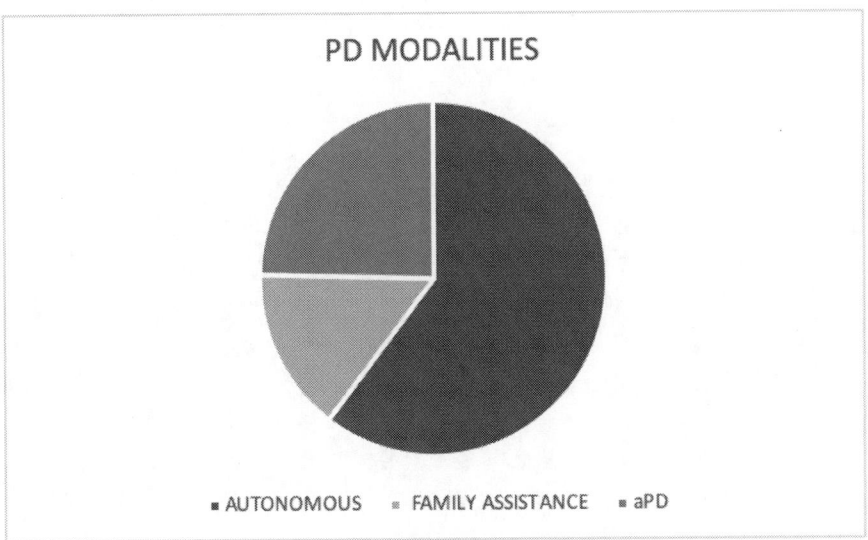

Figure 1. Graphic distribution of the different modalities of peritoneal dialysis in CHU Brugmann since the beginning of the peritoneal dialysis (1996) to juin 2018 (from RDPLF registry).

After consulting the hospital records, which began in June 2010, we have obtained the rates of peritonitis in patients with assisted peritoneal dialysis, expressed in table 1 and figure 2.

Table 1. Rate of peritonitis of patients using the assisted peritoneal dialysis modality since June 2010

Year	Rate of Peritonitis in Assisted Peritoneal Dialysis Compared to the Total Peritoneal Dialysis Patients
2° half of 2010	36,36%
2011	38,01%
2012	29,62%
2013	22,22%
2014	21,42%
2015	0,00%
2016	23,07%
2017	40,00%
1° half of 2018	33,33%

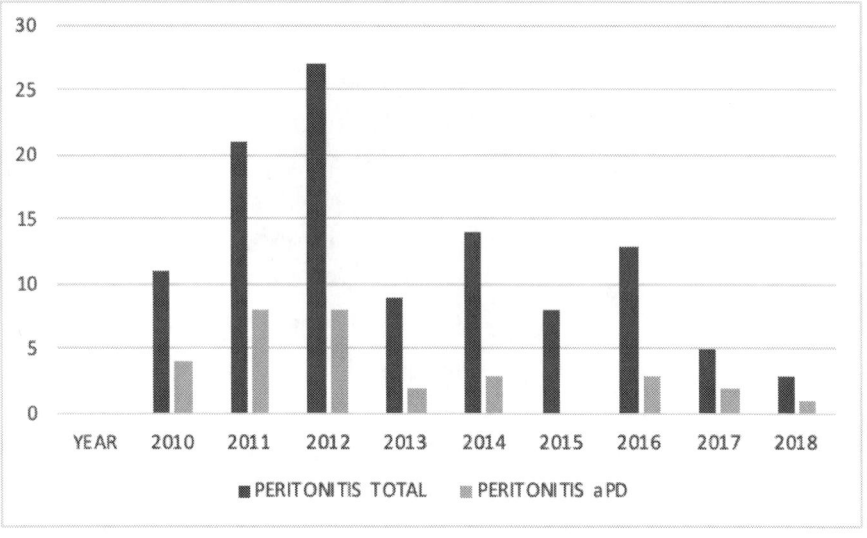

Figure 2. Graphic distribution of the number of peritonitis since the beginning of the registry, the second semester of 2010. aPD: assisted peritoneal dialysis.

In June 2018, the hospital had 22 patients included in the peritoneal dialysis program (21 with Baxter® solutions and only one with Fresenius®).

6 patients out of the total (30%) performed assisted peritoneal dialysis, all of them with Baxter® solutions. Their median age was 61 years (54-66.5). Its demographic, clinical and social characteristics are expressed in table 2.

DISCUSSION

The great number of elderly patients who undergo renal replacement therapy are not candidates for kidney transplantation, so they will undergo lifelong dialysis [9].

Until a few years ago, the only alternative for non-autonomous patients or without family support was in-hospital haemodialysis, which entails a burden that is additional to that of the renal disease itself: transfers to the hospital, need of vascular access, hemodynamic instability linked to the technique...[20-22] Peritoneal dialysis is adequate for them, since it is performed daily, is less aggressive and it is performed at home. The peculiarities of these patients (neurological problems, hearing deficits, problems of strength or ability) make it difficult to perform the technique on their own [20], so the help of the family or specialized personnel who come to their house [9] (assisted peritoneal dialysis) should be considered. This modality, which is used in a growing number of patients, requires a specific funding system to be successful [17], which varies among different countries and health systems. The objective is that it become attractive for care companies and inexpensive for healthcare systems, so its maximum cost should be that of in-hospital haemodialysis [17, 23, 24].

Table 2. Description of the patients receiving assisted peritoneal dialysis in June 2018

Date of Birth	Sex	Main Disease	Debut Dialy-Sis	Technique	Nationality	Type Of Care	N° Peritonitis	Germ
1971	M	HT	2017	APD	MAURITANIA	EVERYTHING*	0	
1934	W	DM	2018	APD	GREECE	ASSEMBLY CYCLER	0	
1950	W	DM	2016	CAPD	VIETNAM	5 DAYS/WEEK	0	
1966	W	DM	2018	APD	CONGO	EVERYTHING**	1	S. sanguinis
1958	W	NK	2010	APD	MOROCCO	ASSEMBLY CYCLER	4	S. haemolyticus S. salivarius Coagulase-negative staphylococcus NOT ISOLATED
1956	M	DM	2016, aPD 2017	APD	BELGIUM	ASSEMBLY CYCLER	1	NOT ISOLATED (before aPD)

aPD: assisted peritoneal dialysis, APD: automatic peritoneal dialysis, CAPD; continuous ambulatory peritoneal dialysis, DM: diabetes mellitus, HT: hypertension, M: Man, NK: not known, W: woman.

* Disabled Patient.

** Depressive Syndrome.

The assisted peritoneal dialysis has several advantages: it offers a home treatment to non-autonomous patients or to patients without family support, it provides a home nurse, who offers psychological support, food training, manages the material, prevents accidents, helps the collection of urine samples and dialyzed for consultations and records the monitoring data: weight, blood pressure, ultrafiltration debit [4]. In addition, the assisted peritoneal dialysis program of this centre allows direct contact between the home staff and the Peritoneal Dialysis Unit in case of problems. This reduces hospitalizations and delays the transfer to nursing homes [19, 23].

In the hospital of our study, 86 patients have chosen this technique, 24.57% of the 350 patients of the peritoneal dialysis program since 1996, a figure who is clearly lower than the autonomous patients, but higher than the patients helped by their family. This underscores the importance of favouring this program to avoid transfer to haemodialysis [24].

These patients are relatively young, with a median age of 66.5 years (60-76.75), with respect to the GFNB statistics (Group of French-speaking Nephrologists of Belgium), which show a median age of 70-80 years [19]. This implies that the assisted peritoneal dialysis, initially designed for elderly patients [20-22], can also be applied to young people, who may have similar limitations to the elderly: physical (disabled), psychological (depressed), and social (immigrants who do not speak the language and suffer from isolation) [23-25]. The latter problem is particularly frequent in the population of CHU Brugmann, as shown by the patients in June 2018: 5 (83.33%) are foreigners with language difficulties and isolation, which makes learning difficult and makes home assistance indispensable [23]. Different studies show a rate of peritonitis in assisted peritoneal dialysis not higher (even lower) than that of patients with autonomy or with family help [26, 27]. Our study confirms this finding: the rate of peritonitis in assisted peritoneal dialysis is within 30% of the total, with a small rate of hospitalizations. This is a consequence of the rigorous protocols and learning conditions imposed by the CHU. In two specific moments (2011 and 2012) the peritonitis increased considerably. This was resolved with the updating of the care protocols and the reinforcement of the training of nurses of the Peritoneal Dialysis Unit of the CHU Brugmann and nurses belonging to the care companies [19].

CONCLUSION

CHU Brugmann assisted peritoneal dialysis program offers peritoneal dialysis to all patients who have no medical contraindications. This philosophy prevents many transfers to haemodialysis and considerably improves the patients' quality of life. The protocols for the training of home-based personnel are very strict, to ensure the correct performance of the technique, the continuity of care in the absence of staff and a low rate of complications, mainly peritonitis. This type of dialysis is particularly attractive in immigrant and in isolated patients (not only in elderly people), who have clear difficulties in order to acquire sufficient autonomy to perform the technique themselves in a correct and safe way.

Our study confirms that assisted peritoneal dialysis is an effective and safe practice, but it needs some strict conditions and a strong planification in order to be successful and to avoid peritonitis and the failure of the technique.

REFERENCES

[1] Fenton S S, Schabubel D E, Desmeules M, Morrison H I, Mao Y, Coppleston P, Jeffery J R, Kjellstrand C M: Hemdialysis versus Peritoneal Dialysis: A comparison of adjusted mortality rates. *Am. J. Kidney Dis.* 1997; 30: 334-342.

[2] Collins A J, Hao W, Xia H, Ebben J P, Everson SE, Constantini E G, Ma J Z: Mortality risks of peritoneal dialysis and hemodialysis. *Am. J. Kidney Dis.* 1999; 34: 1065-1074.

[3] van Esch S, Krediet R T, Struijk D G: 32 years experience of peritoneal dialysis related peritonitis in a university hospital. *Perit. Dial. Int.* 2014; 34: 162-170.

[4] Povlsen J V, Ivarsen P: Assisted automated peritoneal dialysis for the functionally dependent and elderly patient. *Perit. Dial. Int.* 2005; 25: S60-S63.

[5] Li P K, Szeto C C, Piraino B, et al. Peritoneal Dialysis-Related Infections Recommendations: 2010 Update. *Perit. Dial. Int.* 2010;30(4):393-423.

[6] Figueiredo A E, Bernardini J, Bowes E, Hiramatsu M, Price V, Su C, Walker R, Brunier G: A syllabus for teaching peritoneal dialysis to patients and caregivers. *Perit. Dial. Int.* 2016, 36:592-605.

[7] Zhang L, Hawley C M, Johnson D W: Focus on peritoneal dialysis training: Working to decrease peritonitis rates. *Nephrol. Dial. Transplant.* 2016, 31: 214-222, 2016.

[8] Piraino B, Bernardini J, Brown E, et al. ISPD Position Statement on Reducing the Risks of Peritoneal Dialysis Related Infections. *Perit. Dial. Int.* 2011; 31:614-630.

[9] Covic A, Bammens B, Lobbedez T, Segall L, Heimbürger O, van Biesen W, Fouque D, Vanholder R. Educating end-stage renal disease patients on dialysis modality selection: clinical advice from the European Renal Best Practice (ERBP) Advisory Board. *Nephrol. Dial. Transplant.* 2010 Jun;25(6):1757-9.

[10] Johnson D W, Brown F G, Clarke M, Boudville N, Elias T J, Foo M W, Jones B, Kulkarni H, Langham R, Ranganathan D, Schollum J, Suranyi M, Tan SH, Voss: Effects of biocompatible versus standard fluid on peritoneal dialysis outcomes. *J. Am. Soc. Nephrol.* 2012; 23: 1097-1107.

[11] Nessim S J, Nisenbaum R, Bargman J M, et al. Microbiology of peritonitis in peritoneal dialysis patients with multiple episodes. *Perit. Dial. Int.* 2012;32(3):316-21.

[12] Rosman J B, Johnson D W. Enterococcal peritonitis in peritoneal dialysis: the danger from within?. *Perit. Dial. Int.* 2011; 31(5):518-21.

[13] Wiggins K J, Craig J C, Johnson D W, Strippoli G F M. Treatment for peritoneal dialysis-associated peritonitis (Review) *Cochrane Database Syst. Rev.* 2008, 23;(1):CD005284.

[14] Miles R, Hawley C M, McDonald S P, et al. Predictors and outcomes of fungal peritonitis in peritoneal dialysis patients. *Kidney Int.* 2009; 76:622-8.

[15] Ram R, Swarnalatha G, Akpolat T, Dakshinamurty K V. Mycobacterium tuberculous peritonitis in CAPD patients: a report of 11 patients and review of literature. *Int. Urol. Nephrol.* 2013; 45(4):1129-35.

[16] Figueiredo A E, Moraes T P, Bernardini J, Poli-de-Figueiredo C E, Barretti P, Olandoski M, Pecoits-Filho R; BRAZPD Investigators. Impact of patient training patterns on peritonitis rates in a large national cohort study. *Nephrol. Dial. Transplant.* 2015; 30(1):137-42.

[17] Dratwa M. Costs of home assistance for peritoneal dialysis: results of a European survey. *Kidney Int.* 2008;73:S72–5.

[18] RDPLF [Internet]. *Pontoise, France: Registre de Dialyse Péritonéale de Langue Française et hémodialyse.*1988 -[cited 2018 Jun 08]. Available from: http://www.rdplf.org.

[19] Rossez N, Brayer I, Montag M, Poppe A, Dratwa M. La DP assistée en Belgique. Expérience d'un centre. In: *Paper presented in the XIVème Sumposium du RDPLF*. France: Château de Montvillargenne (Gouvieux); 2017. [Assisted PD in Belgium. Experience of a center.]

[20] Béchade C, Lobbedez T, Ivarsen P, Povlsen J V. Assisted Peritoneal Dialysis for Older People with End-Stage Renal Disease: The French and Danish Experience. *Perit. Dial. Int.* 2015 Nov;35(6):663-6.

[21] Brown E A. Should older patients be offered peritoneal dialysis? *Perit. Dial. Int.* 2008; 28:444–8.

[22] Blake P G. Peritoneal dialysis: a "kinder, gentler" treatment for the elderly? (Editorial). *Perit. Dial. Int.* 2008; 28:435–6.

[23] Brown E A, Dratwa M, Povlsen J. Assisted peritoneal dialysis, an evolving dialysis modality. *Nephrol. Dial. Transplant.* 2007; 22:3091–2.

[24] Brown E A, Wilkie M. Assisted Peritoneal Dialysis as an Alternative to In-Center Hemodialysis. *Clin. J. Am. Soc. Nephrol.* 2016 Sep 7; 11(9):1522-4.

[25] Guillouët S, Lobbedez T, Lanot A, Verger C, Ficheux M, Béchade C. Factors associated with nurse assistance among peritoneal dialysis patients: a cohort study from the French Language Peritoneal Dialysis Registry. *Nephrol. Dial. Transplant.* 2017 Dec 25.

[26] Oliver M J, Al-Jaishi A A, Dixon S N, Perl J, Jain A K, Lavoie S D, Nash D M, Paterson J M, Lok C E, Quinn R R. Hospitalization Rates for Patients on Assisted Peritoneal Dialysis Compared with In-Center Hemodialysis. *Clin. J. Am. Soc. Nephrol.* 2016 Sep 7;11(9):1606-14.

[27] Duquennoy S, Béchade C, Verger C, Ficheux M, Ryckelynck J-P, Lobbedez T: Is peritonitis risk increased in elderly patients on peritoneal dialysis? Report from the French Language Peritoneal Dialysis Registry (RDPLF). *Perit. Dial. Int.* 36: 291–296, 2016.

In: Peritonitis
Editor: David F. Walker

ISBN: 978-1-53619-624-5
© 2021 Nova Science Publishers, Inc.

Chapter 3

SECONDARY PERITONITIS: CAUSES, DIAGNOSIS AND TREATMENT

Carlos San Miguel-Méndez, Jaime Ruiz-Tovar[*],
*Ana Minaya-Bravo, Marina Perez-Flecha
and Miguel Angel Garcia-Ureña*
Department of Surgery, Henares University Hospital, Madrid, Spain

ABSTRACT

The peritoneum is a semipermeable membrane that allows a flux of solutes into and from the peritoneal cavity. Peritonitis denotes inflammation of the peritoneum, whose cause is not specific. It mainly exists two different types of this intraabdominal infection: spontaneous bacterial peritonitis (SBP) or secondary peritonitis (SP).

SPB is often presented in cirrhotic patients, in whom altered small intestinal motility and the presence of hypochlorhydria due to the use of proton pump inhibitors predisposes an overgrowth of specific organisms, especially *E. Coli*. They are those processes in which a source of intra-abdominal contamination cannot be evidenced.

---

[*] Corresponding Author's E-mail: jruiztovar@gmail.com.

In SP, the infection is produced by the breakdown of the anatomo-functional barrier of the wall of the gastrointestinal tract or annex glands, with a discharge of septic content into the peritoneal cavity. The main causes are the following: acute appendicitis, diverticulitis, perforated peptic ulcer, intestinal obstruction with strangulation of the small bowel, trauma, pelvic infections and intraoperative contamination. SP is usually polymicrobial, with a predominance of gram-negative bacilli (such as *E. Coli* or *Klebsiella*) and anaerobic organisms (e.g., *Bacteroides fragilis*).

Despite the advances in surgical techniques, antibiotic-therapy and intensive care support; mortality and morbidity remain high, while its management stays difficult and complex.

In this chapter, we will discuss in detail these different types of peritoneum infections, with their principles of diagnosis and last evidence in treatment.

Keywords: spontaneous bacterial peritonitis, secondary peritonitis

INTRODUCTION

The peritoneum is a semipermeable membrane that allows a flux of solutes into and from the peritoneal cavity. Peritonitis denotes inflammation of the peritoneum; whose cause is not specific. This clinically important condition has a wide variety of clinical courses as well as high morbidity and mortality due to secondary multiorgan dysfunction [1]. The key-points to successful treatment are early recognition of the etiologic condition and removal of the causal organism.

Peritonitis has been divided into three different categories depending on the etiology of the disease:

Primary peritonitis results from bacterial translocation, hematogenous spread or the iatrogenic contamination of the abdomen without a macroscopic defect in the gastrointestinal tract [2].

Primary peritonitis usually constitutes spontaneous bacterial peritonitis, which is often presented in cirrhotic patients, in whom altered small intestinal motility and the presence of hypochlorhydria due to the use of proton pump inhibitors predisposes an overgrowth of specific organisms, especially *E. Coli*. It also occurs in infancy and early childhood and immunocompromised hosts. They are those processes in which a source of intra-abdominal contamination cannot be evidenced.

Secondary peritonitis (SP), in contrast, results from the direct contamination of the peritoneum by leakage from the gastrointestinal or urological tracts. Among the main causes of SP, it has been described: acute appendicitis, perforated peptic ulcer, bowel obstruction, perforated hollow viscus, pelvic infections and intraoperative contamination.

Tertiary peritonitis is a less well-defined entity that refers to SP that persists more than 48 hours after an effort of surgical cause control [3]. It is categorized by persistent or recurrent infections with organisms of little virulence or with a tendency for the immunocompromised patient.

It is usually the most delayed and severe consequence of nosocomial intra-abdominal infection and has a high mortality rate of 60% [4].

Peritonitis is also classified either as local or diffuse. Local peritonitis refers to a minor location of the infection, which is usually enclosed or contained by adjoining organs. On the contrary, diffuse or generalized peritonitis means that infection has been spread to the whole abdominal cavity.

SECONDARY PERITONITIS

SP accounts for 1% of urgent or emergent hospital admissions and is the second leading cause of sepsis in patients in intensive care units (ICU) globally. Overall mortality is 6%, but mortality rises to 35% in patients who develop severe sepsis [2]. It depends on patients' age; pre-existing cardiovascular, liver, renal, or neurologic disease; a non-appendicular source of infection; delay in intervention beyond 24 hours; and the extent of peritonitis [5, 6].

Aggressive and prompt surgical intervention is mandatory to deliver optimal care for patients and improve their outcomes.

Epidemiology, Causes and Clinical Presentation

The incidence of SP is difficult to assess. Intra-abdominal infections are found to occur in 25% of patients with multiple organ failure in surgical ICUs [7].

Three large observational studies from the United States and Europe have described the main etiologies and frequencies of SP [5, 6, 8]:

Acute Appendicitis (31-50%)

It is associated with lower mortality, shorter duration of hospital stay, and lower morbidity than other intraabdominal infections [9]. Complicated appendicitis is successfully treated with appendectomy and antibiotic management in up to 90% of cases. Mortality in acute appendicitis has been described as inferior to 1% [10].

Colon (15-32%)

Colonic perforations are the second cause of SP in the Western world, and acute diverticulitis is the most common disease process resulting in a perforation. While most patients with spontaneously perforated diverticulitis require surgery, the choice of techniques depends upon the extent of peritoneal contamination as evaluated by the Hinchey classification system.

In general, the majority of microperforations (not included in the Hinchey classification), Hinchey I, and Hinchey II perforations can be managed nonoperatively, while most Hinchey III and IV perforations require surgical intervention [11].

Perforated colon cancer, ischemic colitis, and foreign body perforations are other causes of SP due to disease of the colon [10].

The reason for typhoidal perforations may be due to poor sanitary condition in developing countries, exposing the patients to Salmonella infection in the community, which may result into perforations [12].

Small Bowel (7-13%)

Small intestine perforations are relatively uncommon as a source of peritonitis in the Western world in contrast to Eastern countries [13]. Most perforations are due to intestinal ischemia or iatrogenic perforations (unrecognized traumatic injuries) [2].

Treatment is resection of the involved segment with primary anastomosis or laparostomy with *second-look* surgery. It means a reoperation 24 to 48 hours after urgent surgery to safely perform a delayed anastomosis whenever possible after resuscitation patient measures in ICU.

Gastroduodenal (8-18%)

Gastroduodenal perforations have decreased significantly in Western countries due to medical treatment of peptic ulcer disease and to prophylaxis for stress ulcers in ICU patients [10].

At the beginning of the XX century, peptic ulcer disease was the most common indication for gastric surgery. Nonetheless, in present it only infrequently requires operation, which is usually performed as a primary closure of perforation without the need of further techniques.

Biliary Tract (1-6%)

It mainly comprised acute cholecystitis processes. Progressive symptoms and signs such as high fever, hemodynamic instability, or pain indicate disease progression, which is a sign of gallbladder gangrene and an indication for emergency cholecystectomy to prevent further complications: perforation and sepsis.

Other Causes

There are also less frequent but also registered iatrogenic causes, such as endoscopic perforations, anastomotic leak, missed enterotomies and infected foreign bodies [2].

Moreover, infections after elective procedures on the gastrointestinal tract or the other abdominal viscera account for 20–25% of patients with peritonitis [9].

Peritonitis usually presents as an acute abdomen. Local findings include generalized abdominal tenderness, rigidity, abdominal distension and decreased bowel sounds. Systemic findings include fever with chills or rigor, restlessness, tachycardia, tachypnea, dehydration, oliguria, disorientation and ultimately shock [14].

Severity Classifications

Despite advances in surgical techniques, antimicrobial therapy, and ICU support; the management of SP continues to be highly challenging and complex [12]. Early prognostic evaluation of SP is desirable to provide an objective classification of the severity of the disease and select high risk patients for more aggressive therapeutic procedures [15, 16].

It is usually assessed by the Acute Physiologic and Chronic Health Evaluation (APACHE) scoring system, of which there are four versions (APACHE I through IV) [17, 18]. Even though this is not a specific peritonitis score.

Mannheim Peritonitis Index (MPI) predicts the short-term risk of mortality of a patient with peritonitis. It has the advantage that it can be calculated during operation whereas APACHE-IV, the latest version, uses 129 variables derived from the worst values from the initial 24 hours of ICU admission [19].

Another predictive scoring system is the Sequential Organ Failure Assessment (SOFA) score. It was designed to evaluate the severity of organ dysfunction in patients who were critically ill from sepsis. It uses simple data of organ function to estimate a severity score. It is calculated 24 hours after admission and every 48 hours subsequently. The mean and the highest scores are most predictive of mortality [20].

Diagnosis

Physical Examination

It is mandatory for an initial examination to determine whether patients are unstable or not. If patients do not present with signs of instability, they will be presumable candidates for CT scan further diagnosis. On the contrary, if patients present altered vital signs and worst appearance (hemodynamic instability), they will be probably conducted to urgent surgery.

During anamnesis, it is relevant to define the timing, location, and character of the pain, along with concomitant symptoms as well as to establish the magnitude of peritonitis. Localized will present with peritoneal signs limited to one or two abdominal quadrants instead of diffused peritonitis, with rigidity, rebound tenderness, or guarding in the whole abdomen [2].

Older and obese patients are particularly challenging, as the physical examination may be unpredictable [21–23].

Laboratory Tests

Laboratory testing has a well-established role in the diagnosis of a wide range of acute abdominal pathologies. Conversely, their position in the initial management of SP is limited.

- White blood cell (WBC): The elevation of WBC usually represents bacterial infection. However, its augmentation does not correspond to specific infections. Leucocytosis is present in physiologic stress reactions, after doing intense sports activities or in pregnancy [24]. Therefore, WBC has not been used as a diagnostic tool or a prognostic factor in SP [25].
- Lactate: It has been studied extensively as a marker of systemic hypoperfusion and is independently associated with mortality in surgical patients with sepsis [2, 26, 27].
- Others: C reactive protein and procalcitonin are proteins that could be elevated during SP. C reactive protein has been related to septic

complications in patients already operated [28–30] and procalcitonin has more specificity for a bacterial infection rather than others [31, 32].

Imaging

Patients with generalized peritonitis or localized peritonitis with hemodynamic instability do not need imaging, as this would not alter the need for urgent surgery [2]. However, in stable patients with localized peritonitis, imaging is essential to evaluate the magnitude of contamination.

To date, multidetector CT represents the best imaging modality to evaluate patients with acute abdominal pain [33]. Although CT is the most sensitive imaging investigation for detecting urgent conditions in patients with abdominal pain, using ultrasonography first and CT only in those with negative or inconclusive ultrasonography results in the best sensitivity and lowers exposure to radiation [34].

Treatment

Inflammation related to SP associates a significant and mainly compartmentalized peritoneal cytokine reaction that reveals the gravity and prognosis of the disease. Current surgical and antibiotic therapy can clear the peritoneal cavity of infection, but patients continue to die of uncontrolled activation of the inflammatory cascade produced [35]. Therefore, suitable treatment should be delivered promptly to these patients.

The principles of management of SP are fluid resuscitation, the use of empiric antibiotics, and control of the septic focus [2].

Firstly, treatment should be preceded by designation to patients to some severity score during clinical triaging, as APACHE, MPI or SOFA, among others. It will be essential to confirm the posterior effectiveness of treatments, as well as to inform patients and their relatives with greater objectivity [36].

Resuscitation

Resuscitation involves all measures to preserve or enhance organ perfusion and oxygenation. Suitable resuscitation within 6 hours of the onset of sepsis increases survival [37].

Antimicrobial Therapy

International guidelines have recently assessed the selection of proper antibiotic treatment in SP patients [38]. Patients with SP should be treated empirically with broad-spectrum antibiotics including Gram-positive, Gram-negative, and anaerobic coverage.

Delay in the administration of antibiotics after diagnosing SP rises death rates with an odds ratio of 1.021 (95% CI: 1.003–1.038) [39]. However, even the benefit of early empiric antimicrobial coverage has been demonstrated, regimens must be adjusted when culture results become available [40].

A substantial amount of SP patients who are admitted to the ICU presents colonization with yeasts and fungal strains, mainly Candida [37]. Empiric fungal treatment should be added in patients at high risks, such as patients with recurrent abdominal surgery or SP due to anastomotic leaks [41, 42].

After initial management, persistent clinical signs of fever or leukocytosis should prompt a search for a drainable focus of infection in the abdomen or treatable site elsewhere [7].

Surgical Treatment

Patients with a localized intraabdominal abscess are often candidates for percutaneous drainage, which is usually performed under CT or ultrasound guidance [10]. Routine culture of the sites of infection seems worthwhile and empirical therapy should be as comprehensive as possible and should cover all potential pathogens [7].

Patients with more complex abscesses, associated necrotic tissue, or who require resection of a neoplasm are usually better candidates for open drainage and consequently for urgent laparotomy.

Lack of improvement in mild peritonitis operated patients determines the necessity for a relaparotomy, referred to as the *on-demand* strategy [43]. In contrast, severe peritonitis patients usually need more aggressive surgical treatments, such as radical peritoneal debridement, "open abdomen" treatment, and planned relaparotomy strategy [37]. More recently, it has been described *damage control surgery*. It is a trauma principle where the open abdomen is temporarily closed with a mesh inlay and negative pressure wound therapy added. Delayed abdominal closure is contemplated but not always achieved.

There is evidence that multiple relaparotomies increase the systemic inflammatory mediator response rising in increased incidence of mortality [44].

The treatment of SP demands a multidisciplinary approach, where surgeons, radiologists and intensivists must work together with a close availability. Approximately 40% of all patients diagnosed with SP will need ICU admission [37]. Thus, prompt elimination of the infectious focus with surgery when needed, intensive resuscitation and antimicrobial therapy are cornerstones in the treatment of SP.

REFERENCES

[1] Ragetly, GR; Bennett, RA; Ragetly, CA. Ätiologie, Pathophysiologie und Diagnose der septischen Peritonitis. *Tierärztliche Prax Ausgabe K Kleintiere/Heimtiere*, 2012, Jan 6, 40(04), 290–7. [Pathophysiology and diagnosis of septic peritonitis. *Veterinary practice issue K small animals / pets*]

[2] Ross, JT; Matthay, MA; Harris, HW. Secondary peritonitis: principles of diagnosis and intervention. *BMJ*, 2018, Jun 18, 361, k1407.

[3] Ordoñez, CA; Puyana, JC. Management of Peritonitis in the Critically Ill Patient. *Surg Clin North Am*, 2006 Dec, 86(6), 1323–49.

[4] Martín-López, A; Castaño-Ávila, S; Maynar-Moliner, FJ; Urturi-Matos, JA; Manzano-Ramírez, A; Martín-López, HP. Peritonitis

terciaria: tan difícil de definir como de tratar. *Cir Esp*, 2012 Jan, 90(1), 11–6. [Tertiary peritonitis: as difficult to define as it is to treat.]

[5] Anaya, DA; Nathens, AB. Risk Factors for Severe Sepsis in Secondary Peritonitis. *Surg Infect* (Larchmt), 2003 Dec, 4(4), 355–62.

[6] Sartelli, M; Catena, F; Ansaloni, L; Leppaniemi, A; Taviloglu, K; van Goor, H; et al. Complicated intra-abdominal infections in Europe: a comprehensive review of the CIAO study. *World J Emerg Surg*, 2012, 7(1), 36.

[7] Holzheimer, aarg; Mannick, JA. Surgical Treatment. Evidence-based and Problem-oriented. *Eur J Surg.*, 2002, 168, 310.

[8] Gauzit, R; Péan, Y; Barth, X; Mistretta, F; Lalaude, O. Epidemiology, Management, and Prognosis of Secondary Non-Postoperative Peritonitis: A French Prospective Observational Multicenter Study. *Surg Infect* (Larchmt), 2009 Apr, 10(2), 119–27.

[9] Merlino, JI; Malangoni, MA; Smith, CM; Lange, RL. Prospective Randomized Trials Affect the Outcomes of Intraabdominal Infection. *Ann Surg*, 2001 Jun, 233(6), 859–66.

[10] Malangoni, MA; Inui, T. Peritonitis - The Western experience. *World J Emerg Surg*, 2006, 1, 25.

[11] Hinchey, EJ; Schaal, PG; Richards, GK. Treatment of perforated diverticular disease of the colon. *Adv Surg*, 1978, 12, 85–109.

[12] Mabewa, A; Seni, J; Chalya, PL; Mshana, SE; Gilyoma, JM. Etiology, treatment outcome and prognostic factors among patients with secondary peritonitis at Bugando Medical Centre, Mwanza, Tanzania. *World J Emerg Surg*, 2015, Dec 6, 10(1), 47.

[13] Gupta, S; Kaushik, R. Peritonitis - The Eastern experience. *World J Emerg Surg*, 2006, 1, 13.

[14] Mabewa, A; Seni, J; Chalya, PL; Mshana, SE; Gilyoma, JM. Etiology, treatment outcome and prognostic factors among patients with secondary peritonitis at Bugando Medical Centre, Mwanza, Tanzania. *World J Emerg Surg*, 2015, Dec 6, 10(1), 47.

[15] Sharma, S; Kaneria, R; Sharma, A; Khare, A. Perforation peritonitis: a clinical study regarding etiology, clinical presentation and management strategies. *Int Surg J*, 2019, Nov 26, 6(12), 4455.

[16] Billing, A; Fröhlich, D. Prediction of outcome using the Mannheim peritonitis index in 2003 patients. *Br J Surg*, 1994 Feb, 81(2), 209–13.

[17] Bhattacharya, A; Singh, R; Vajifdar, H; Kumar, N. Preoperative predictors of mortality in adult patients with perforation peritonitis. *Indian J Crit Care Med*, 2011 Jul, 15(3), 157–63.

[18] Knaus, WA; Wagner, DP; Draper, EA; Zimmerman, JE; Bergner, M; Bastos, PG; et al. The APACHE III Prognostic System. *Chest*, 1991 Dec, 100(6), 1619–36.

[19] Zimmerman, JE; Kramer, AA; McNair, DS; Malila, FM. Acute Physiology and Chronic Health Evaluation (APACHE) IV: Hospital mortality assessment for today's critically ill patients*. *Crit Care Med*, 2006 May, 34(5), 1297–310.

[20] Sharma, S; Singh, S; Makkar, N; Kumar, A; Sandhu, M. Assessment of severity of peritonitis using mannheim peritonitis index. *Niger J Surg*, 2016, 22(2), 118.

[21] Ferreira, FL; Bota, DP; Bross, A; Mélot, C; Vincent, JL. Serial evaluation of the SOFA score to predict outcome in critically ill patients. *JAMA*, 2001, Oct 10, 286(14), 1754–8.

[22] Wroblewski, M; Mikulowski, P. Peritonitis in Geriatric Inpatients. *Age Ageing*, 1991, 20(2), 90–4.

[23] Ragsdale, L; Southerland, L. Acute Abdominal Pain in the Older Adult. *Emerg Med Clin North Am*, 2011 May, 29(2), 429–48.

[24] Edwards, ED; Jacob, BP; Gagner, M; Pomp, A. Presentation and Management of Common Post–Weight Loss Surgery Problems in the Emergency Department. *Ann Emerg Med*, 2006 Feb, 47(2), 160–6.

[25] Cerny, J; Rosmarin, AG. Why Does My Patient Have Leukocytosis? *Hematol Oncol Clin North Am*, 2012 Apr, 26(2), 303–19.

[26] Solomkin, JS; Mazuski, JE; Bradley, JS; Rodvold, KA; Goldstein, EJC; Baron, EJ; et al. Diagnosis and management of complicated

intra-abdominal infection in adults and children (IDSA guidelines). *Clin Infect Dis.*, 2010, 11, 79-109.

[27] Bakker, J; de Lima, AP. Increased blood lacate levels: an important warning signal in surgical practice. *Crit Care*, 2004 Apr, 8(2), 96–8.

[28] Moore, LJ; McKinley, BA; Turner, KL; Todd, SR; Sucher, JF; Valdivia, A; et al. The Epidemiology of Sepsis in General Surgery Patients. *J Trauma Int Infect Crit Care*, 2011 Mar, 70(3), 672–80.

[29] Ortega-Deballon, P; Radais, F; Facy, O; D'Athis, P; Masson, D; Charles PE; et al. C-Reactive Protein Is an Early Predictor of Septic Complications After Elective Colorectal Surgery. *World J Surg*, 2010, Apr 5, 34(4), 808–14.

[30] Almeida, AB; Faria, G; Moreira, H; Pinto-de-Sousa, J; Correia-da-Silva, P; Maia, JC. Elevated serum C-reactive protein as a predictive factor for anastomotic leakage in colorectal surgery. *Int J Surg*, 2012, 10(2), 87–91.

[31] Scepanovic, MS; Kovacevic, B; Cijan, V; Antic, A; Petrovic, Z; Asceric, R; et al. C-reactive protein as an early predictor for anastomotic leakage in elective abdominal surgery. *Tech Coloproctol*, 2013, Oct 26, 17(5), 541–7.

[32] Cosse, C; Regimbeau, JM; Fuks, D; Mauvais, F; Scotte, M. Serum Procalcitonin for Predicting the Failure of Conservative Management and the Need for Bowel Resection in Patients with Small Bowel Obstruction. *J Am Coll Surg*, 2013 May, 216(5), 997–1004.

[33] Markogiannakis, H; Memos, N; Messaris, E; Dardamanis, D; Larentzakis, A; Papanikolaou, D; et al. Predictive value of procalcitonin for bowel ischemia and necrosis in bowel obstruction. *Surgery*, 2011 Mar, 149(3), 394–403.

[34] Filippone, A; Cianci, R; Pizzi, AD; Esposito, G; Pulsone, P; Tavoletta, A; et al. CT findings in acute peritonitis: a pattern-based approach. *Diagnostic Interv Radiol*, 2015, Oct 15, 21(6), 435–40.

[35] Lameris, W; van Randen, A; van Es, HW; van Heesewijk, JPM; van Ramshorst, B; Bouma, WH; et al. Imaging strategies for detection of urgent conditions in patients with acute abdominal pain: diagnostic accuracy study. *BMJ*, 2009, Jun 26, 338(jun26 2), b2431–b2431.

[36] Shein, M; Wittmann, DH; Holzheimer, R; Condon, RE. Hypothesis: Compartmentalization of cytokines in intraabdominal infection. *Surgery*, 1996 Jun, 119(6), 694–700.

[37] Cavallaro, A; Catania, V; Cavallaro, M; Zanghì, A; Cappellani, A. Management of secondary peritonitis: our experience. *Ann Ital Chir*, 2008, 79(4), 255–60.

[38] van Ruler, O; Boermeester, MA. Surgical treatment of secondary peritonitis: A continuing problem. *Chirurg*, 2017 Jan, 88(Suppl 1), 1–6.

[39] Montravers, P; Blot, S; Dimopoulos, G; Eckmann, C; Eggimann, P; Guirao, X; et al. Therapeutic management of peritonitis: a comprehensive guide for intensivists. *Intensive Care Med*, 2016, Aug 16, 42(8), 1234–47.

[40] Barie, PS; Hydo, LJ; Shou, J; Larone, DH; Eachempati, SR. Influence of Antibiotic Therapy on Mortality of Critical Surgical Illness Caused or Complicated by Infection. *Surg Infect* (Larchmt), 2005 Mar, 6(1), 41–54.

[41] van Ruler, O; Kiewiet, JJS; van Ketel, RJ; Boermeester, MA. Initial microbial spectrum in severe secondary peritonitis and relevance for treatment. *Eur J Clin Microbiol Infect Dis*, 2012, May 29, 31(5), 671–82.

[42] Montravers, P; Dupont, H; Eggimann, P. Intra-abdominal candidiasis: the guidelines-forgotten non-candidemic invasive candidiasis. *Intensive Care Med*, 2013 Dec, 39(12), 2226–30.

[43] Bassetti, M; Marchetti, M; Chakrabarti, A; Colizza, S; Garnacho-Montero, J; Kett, DH; et al. A research agenda on the management of intra-abdominal candidiasis: results from a consensus of multinational experts. *Intensive Care Med*, 2013, Dec 9, 39(12), 2092–106.

[44] van Ruler, O; Mahler, CW; Boer, KR; Reuland, EA; Gooszen, HG; Opmeer, BC; et al. Comparison of On-Demand vs Planned Relaparotomy Strategy in Patients With Severe Peritonitis. *JAMA*, 2007, Aug 22, 298(8), 865.

[45] Zugel, N. Circulating Mediators and Organ Function in Patients Undergoing Planned Relaparotomy vs Conventional Surgical Therapy in Severe Secondary Peritonitis. *Arch Surg*, 2002, May 1, 137(5), 590–9.

INDEX

A

abdominal sepsis, 3, 4, 6, 31, 32, 36, 57, 59, 60, 62, 63, 64
acute appendicitis, x, 88, 89, 90
acute respiratory distress syndrome, 33
adults, 26, 61, 62, 66, 99
age, viii, 3, 12, 14, 15, 17, 47, 53, 54, 56, 77, 79, 81, 89
anastomosis, viii, 2, 9, 18, 46, 49, 50, 53, 54, 55, 91
anesthesiologist, 40
antibiotic resistance, 30
antibiotics, 4, 13, 18, 19, 20, 26, 31, 32, 43, 44, 62, 73, 94, 95
antimicrobial therapy, 32, 44, 92, 96
appendicitis, x, 88, 89, 90
assisted peritoneal dialysis, v, vii, ix, 70, 73, 74, 75, 77, 78, 79, 80, 81, 82, 84, 85
auscultation, 11, 16

B

bacteremia, 62
bacteria, 4, 9, 19, 30, 73

bacterial infection, 93, 94
blood, 9, 17, 25, 26, 27, 34, 35, 36, 38, 41, 44, 71, 81, 93, 99
blood circulation, 25, 36
blood cultures, 27
blood flow, 38
blood pressure, 17, 81
blood supply, 9
bowel, x, 42, 88, 89, 92, 99
bowel obstruction, 89, 99

C

carcinoma, 48, 49, 50
cardiac arrest, 38
cardiac output, 17
cardiovascular system, 14
catheter, 17, 26, 27, 70, 71, 72, 73, 76
central nervous system, 14, 36
children, 62, 66, 99
cholecystectomy, 50, 52, 91
chronic kidney disease, 48, 50
circulation, 19, 37, 44
classification, vii, 2, 14, 90, 92
clinical assessment, 6, 12, 32
clinical presentation, 98

closure, 21, 22, 25, 28, 29, 36, 38, 45, 46, 58, 63, 67, 91, 96
colon, 15, 26, 44, 48, 90, 97
compartment syndrome, viii, 2, 20, 29, 33, 35, 36, 46, 64
compliance, 34, 76
complications, viii, ix, 2, 4, 12, 13, 16, 22, 25, 29, 34, 35, 36, 38, 40, 41, 42, 44, 45, 55, 69, 74, 82, 91, 94
contamination, x, 4, 6, 7, 8, 14, 19, 27, 48, 71, 87, 88, 89, 90, 94
cross-sectional study, 74, 75

D

dehydration, 10, 40, 41, 92
dialysis, vii, ix, 48, 49, 69, 70, 71, 72, 73, 74, 75, 76, 77, 78, 79, 80, 81, 82, 83, 84, 85
disease progression, 91
distribution, 28, 30, 31, 45, 77, 78
diverticulitis, x, 50, 51, 88, 90
drainage, 20, 22, 25, 40, 50, 51, 52, 53, 54, 55, 95

E

E. Coli, x, 87, 88
edema, 11, 12, 21, 33, 36
electrolyte, 29, 34, 40, 43, 44, 46
emergency, 14, 25, 28, 38, 47, 48, 49, 91
endotracheal intubation, 17
end-stage renal disease, 83
environment, 29, 75, 76
etiology, viii, 2, 14, 30, 48, 88, 98
evacuation, 20, 25, 27, 28, 51, 52, 54
examinations, 12, 32
excretion, 17, 26, 27, 33, 34, 41, 44
exudate, 3, 4, 14, 22, 25, 28, 36

F

family members, 73, 76, 77
family support, ix, 70, 79, 81
fever, 10, 60, 91, 92, 95
fistulas, 21, 29, 35, 46, 65, 66, 67
fluid, 11, 12, 17, 20, 29, 36, 37, 44, 71, 72, 83, 94
fluid balance, 37
formation, viii, 2, 9, 21, 29, 40, 46, 73
fungal infection, 18, 33, 44, 73

G

gastroenterologist, 40
gastrointestinal tract, x, 4, 30, 37, 39, 88, 91

H

healing, 8, 25, 55, 65, 67
health, 48, 73, 79
health care, 48, 73
health care professionals, 73
heart failure, 38
heart rate, 13
hemodialysis, ix, 38, 69, 70, 71, 72, 73, 74, 82
hemodynamic instability, 79, 94
hemoglobin, 19, 20, 26, 34
hepatic failure, 32
home care agencies, 76
home care services, 74, 77
hydrocortisone, 26, 33
hypertension, 25, 28, 29, 36, 46, 64, 80
hypotension, 5, 10, 26, 37
hypovolemia, 17, 29, 37, 38, 41
hypoxemia, 26, 37

Index

I

iatrogenic, viii, 2, 6, 9, 50, 88, 91
identification, ix, 3, 25, 27, 32, 33, 42
ileostomy, 53, 54
ileum, 26, 44, 49, 53
imaging, vii, 2, 3, 12, 32, 45, 94, 99
immune response, 34
immunocompromised, 89
immunosuppression, 13, 15
infection, ix, x, 3, 4, 6, 7, 8, 10, 13, 18, 19, 20, 21, 25, 27, 29, 30, 31, 32, 33, 42, 44, 46, 48, 55, 56, 59, 60, 61, 62, 66, 71, 72, 87, 88, 89, 90, 94, 95, 99, 100
inflammation, vii, ix, 13, 19, 28, 42, 87, 88
intensive care, vii, x, 1, 2, 3, 4, 12, 13, 14, 17, 25, 29, 32, 33, 35, 47, 57, 58, 60, 61, 62, 64, 88, 89, 100
intensive care unit, 57, 58, 60, 61, 89
intervention, 18, 27, 28, 46, 55, 89, 96
intestinal obstruction, x, 15, 46, 88
intestine, 45, 50, 53, 91
intoxication, 32, 40
intraoperative contamination, x, 4, 88, 89
ischemia, 5, 7, 36, 91, 99

K

kidney, ix, 69, 70, 79
kidney transplantation, 79

L

laparoscopic cholecystectomy, 50, 55
laparostomy, viii, 2, 3, 22, 23, 24, 28, 29, 38, 40, 53, 55, 56, 91
laparotomy, 6, 7, 10, 16, 28, 38, 53, 55, 64, 95

M

management, vii, viii, x, 2, 3, 22, 28, 44, 46, 55, 58, 59, 60, 62, 63, 64, 65, 66, 67, 76, 88, 90, 92, 93, 94, 95, 98, 100
mean arterial pressure, 26, 33, 44
mechanical ventilation, 12, 17, 21, 22, 38
median, 28, 75, 77, 79, 81
medical, viii, 2, 31, 45, 75, 76, 82, 91
medical history, 31, 45
medical science, viii, 2
metabolic disorder, 44
metabolic disturbances, 28, 41
microorganisms, 5, 18, 30, 32, 72
morbidity, vii, ix, x, 1, 3, 4, 12, 14, 39, 42, 56, 71, 88, 90
mortality, vii, viii, ix, x, 1, 2, 3, 4, 5, 6, 12, 15, 22, 32, 36, 38, 42, 56, 57, 61, 62, 65, 71, 82, 88, 89, 90, 92, 93, 96, 98
mortality rate, viii, 2, 22, 82, 89

N

nasogastric tube, 5, 10, 27, 38
necrosis, 21, 28, 50, 99
necrotizing fasciitis, 28
nurses, ix, 70, 73, 74, 75, 76, 82
nursing, 74, 81
nursing home, 74, 81
nutrition, 10, 34, 35, 43, 44
nutritional state, 8, 43, 46

O

organ, 6, 8, 11, 12, 13, 14, 21, 28, 31, 36, 37, 38, 40, 41, 49, 55, 56, 61, 90, 92, 95
organism, 10, 16, 18, 36, 41, 72, 88
oxygen, 15, 17, 26, 33, 44

P

pain, 5, 10, 16, 34, 38, 71, 72, 73, 91, 93, 94, 99
pancreatitis, viii, 2, 8, 48, 50, 52, 53, 55
pathogens, viii, 2, 27, 30, 31, 32, 95
pathology, 5, 39, 47, 49
pathophysiological, 31, 41, 64
pelvic infections, x, 88, 89
peptic ulcer, x, 61, 88, 89, 91
peptic ulcer disease, 91
perforated peptic ulcer, x, 88, 89
perforation, 8, 48, 49, 50, 59, 61, 72, 90, 91, 98
peritoneal cavity, viii, ix, x, 2, 18, 19, 20, 22, 40, 48, 55, 56, 60, 70, 71, 87, 88, 94
peritoneal dialysis, ix, 48, 49, 69, 70, 71, 72, 73, 74, 75, 76, 77, 78, 80, 81, 82, 83, 84, 85
peritoneal lavage, 50, 60
peritoneum, vii, ix, x, 3, 4, 5, 12, 48, 73, 87, 88, 89
peritonitis, v, vii, viii, ix, x, 2, 3, 4, 5, 6, 7, 8, 9, 10, 11, 13, 14, 15, 16, 18, 19, 20, 21, 22, 23, 25, 26, 28, 29, 30, 31, 32, 36, 41, 42, 47, 48, 49, 50, 51, 52, 53, 54, 55, 56, 57, 58, 59, 60, 61, 69, 70, 71, 72, 73, 74, 75, 76, 77, 78, 80, 81, 82, 83, 84, 85, 87, 88, 89, 91, 92, 93, 94, 96, 97, 98, 99, 100, 101
poor performance, viii, 3, 56
population, 46, 75, 81
postoperative peritonitis, v, vii, 1, 2, 3, 4, 5, 7, 9, 10, 11, 16, 17, 21, 23, 35, 47, 48, 50, 52, 53, 54, 55, 56, 57, 58, 60, 97
preparation, iv, viii, 2, 25, 27, 31, 46
prevention, 35, 55, 70, 73
prevention of infection, 70
principles, vii, x, 25, 30, 55, 56, 65, 88, 94, 96
prognosis, 5, 6, 13, 15, 42, 94
proteolytic enzyme, 9, 41, 42
proton pump inhibitors, x, 35, 43, 87, 88
Pseudomonas aeruginosa, 31

R

randomized controlled clinical trials, 57
recovery, 10, 16, 17, 22, 25, 44, 47
relaparotomy, viii, 2, 3, 4, 6, 8, 29, 48, 50, 51, 52, 53, 54, 55, 56, 57, 58, 59, 96, 101
renal replacement therapy, 38, 79
response, ix, 3, 10, 11, 13, 19, 32, 52, 55, 59, 71, 96

S

secondary peritonitis, v, x, 4, 5, 57, 58, 61, 87, 88, 89, 97, 100, 101
sensitivity, 5, 15, 18, 30, 31, 33, 94
sepsis, 3, 4, 5, 6, 11, 12, 13, 14, 17, 25, 26, 29, 30, 31, 32, 36, 42, 43, 44, 52, 53, 54, 55, 56, 57, 58, 59, 60, 62, 63, 66, 89, 91, 92, 93, 95
septic shock, 13, 17, 26, 27, 28, 33, 34, 43, 66
skin, 24, 39, 42, 43, 45, 46
small intestine, 41, 48, 51, 53
spontaneous bacterial peritonitis, x, 87, 88
surgical intervention, 4, 13, 27, 28, 38, 43, 45, 47, 48, 49, 89, 90
surgical techniques, x, 88, 92
surgical treatment, 27, 28, 30, 43, 45, 59, 95, 96, 97
suture, 8, 16, 19, 20, 28, 49, 50
swelling, 5, 10, 11, 12, 16
symptoms, vii, 2, 6, 9, 16, 32, 36, 37, 71, 91, 93
syndrome, 10, 11, 21, 36, 38, 42, 44, 46, 50, 52, 53
systolic blood pressure, 14

T

tactics, viii, 2, 28, 42, 45, 46, 55, 56
therapy, viii, ix, 3, 4, 5, 10, 17, 23, 24, 25, 26, 27, 28, 29, 30, 31, 32, 33, 35, 36, 37, 42, 43, 47, 57, 60, 72, 73, 94, 95, 96
thrombocytopenia, 34
tissue, 9, 17, 25, 26, 29, 95
tissue perfusion, 26
total parenteral nutrition, 44
training, ix, 70, 74, 76, 81, 82, 83, 84
training protocol, ix, 70, 74
treatment, vii, viii, ix, x, 2, 3, 12, 13, 16, 20, 22, 25, 27, 28, 29, 30, 31, 32, 34, 35, 37, 38, 40, 42, 43, 44, 45, 46, 55, 56, 58, 59, 60, 66, 69, 70, 71, 72, 73, 74, 81, 84, 88, 91, 94, 95, 96, 97, 100

U

ultrasonography, 94
ultrasound, 12, 72, 95
urinary bladder, 37, 46
urine, 17, 26, 27, 33, 34, 41, 44, 71, 76, 81

V

ventilation, 33, 37
viscera, viii, 2, 72, 91
visiting nursing staff, 74

W

wound dehiscence, 9, 67
wound infection, viii, 2, 41